Ethics, law and nursing

MANCHESTER
UNIVERSITY PRESS

Ethics, law and nursing

Nina Fletcher and **Janet Holt**

Consultant editors
Margaret Brazier and John Harris

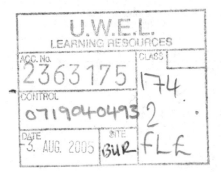
Manchester University Press
Manchester and New York
Distributed exclusively in the USA by Palgrave

Copyright © Nina Fletcher and Janet Holt 1995
Introduction copyright © Margaret Brazier and John Harris 1995

Published by Manchester University Press
Oxford Road, Manchester M13 9NR, UK
and Room 400, 175 Fifth Avenue, New York, NY 10010, USA
http://www.manchesteruniversitypress.co.uk

Distributed exclusively in the USA by
Palgrave, 175 Fifth Avenue, New York, NY 10010, USA

Distributed exclusively in Canada by
UBC Press, University of British Columbia, 2029 West Mall,
Vancouver, BC, Canada V6T 1Z2

British Library Cataloguing-in-Publication Data
A catalogue record for this book is available from the British Library

Library of Congress Cataloging-in-Publication Data

Fletcher, Nina.
    Ethics, law, and nursing / Nina Fletcher and Janet Holt :
consultant editors, Margaret Brazier and John Harris.
        p.   cm.
    ISBN 0–7190–4049–3 (hard). — ISBN 0–7190–4050–7 (pbk.)
    1. Nursing—Law and legislation—Great Britain.   2. Nursing
ethics—Great Britain.   I. Holt, Janet.   II. Title.
KD2968.NBF58   1995
174'.2—dc20   94–27746
                                                            CIP

ISBN 0 7190 4049 3 *hardback*
     0 7190 4050 7 *paperback*

Reprinted in paperback 1996, 1999, 2001

Printed in Great Britain by
Redwood Books, Trowbridge

Contents

Foreword

The Centre for Social Ethics and Policy was established in the University of Manchester in 1986. Since 1989 the Centre has been involved in devising, and initially delivering, courses on ethics and law for nursing students, and organising seminars for nurse practitioners. This book is the result of that experience. We have sought to integrate ethical and legal debate and to explore the complex relationship between ethics and law in nursing practice. We do not offer pre-packaged answers to ethical dilemmas but hope to provoke independent thought and judgment on the part of our readers whether they are students or practitioners. We hope too to stimulate an interest in the subject-matter of the book which can be pursued through the further reading which we recommend at the end of the work.

The first draft of several chapters of the text was prepared by Janet Holt and Nina Fletcher. Both were originally working within the Centre. Janet Holt is both a nurse and a philosophy graduate. Nina Fletcher is a law graduate now lecturing in health care law. We discussed the material with them at each stage and ultimately edited (and to some extent altered) the initial draft. We thank them for their infinite patience with us. We made a collective (if not entirely democratic) decision to dispense with the usual footnotes or references, and sources are acknowledged in the sources and further reading list at the end of the book. We did so to improve the book's readability as it is designed to be picked up and read, if not as a whole, at least in large chunks.

Collaboration is never easy. Those preparing this book come from three very diverse disciplines. Our individual 'philosophies' differ quite radically. We hope that the end result will enable readers to widen their own perspectives on ethical debate in the context of nursing practice. We will be interested in any answers the reader can offer.

Margaret Brazier
John Harris

Table of cases

Note: for brackets, the style of the individual publication has been followed.

A
A. G. v. *Guardian Newspapers (No. 2)* [1988] 3 All ER 545
Airedale NHS Trust v. *Bland* [1993] 1 All ER 859 HL
Allan v. *New Mount Sinai Hospital* (1980) 109 DLR (3d) 536

B
B, Re (a minor) (wardship: medical treatment) [1981] 1 WLR 1421
B, Re (a minor) (wardship: sterilisation) [1987] 2 All ER 206
Barnett v. *Chelsea and Kensington Hospital Management* [1969] 1 QB
  428
Blyth v. *Bloomsbury Area Health Authority* (1985) *The Times*, 24 May,
  (1987) *The Times*, 11 February
Bolam v. *Friern Hospital Management Committee* [1957] 2 All ER 118

C
C, Re (wardship: medical treatment) [1989] 2 All ER 782 CA
C, Re [1994] 1 WLR 290
Callanan v. *Surrey Area Health Authority* [1980] Feb 5 COIT 994/36
Canterbury v. *Spence* (1972) 464 F. 2d 772
Chatterton v. *Gerson* [1981] 3 WLR 1003

D
D, Re (a minor) (wardship: sterilisation) [1976] 1 All ER 326
Devi v. *West Midlands Area Health Authority* [1980] 7 CL 44

E
Emeh v. *Kensington and Chelsea Area Health Authority* [1985] 3 All ER
  1044 CA

Table of statutes

Abortion Act 1967
Access to Health Records Act 1990
Animals (Scientific Procedures) Act 1986
Children Act 1989
Children and Young Persons Act 1933
Congenital Disabilities (Civil Liability) Act 1976
Criminal Law Act 1967
Data Protection Act 1984
European Communities Act 1972
Family Law Reform Act 1969
Hospital Complaints Procedures Act 1985
Human Fertilisation and Embryology Act 1990
Medicines Act 1968
Mental Health Act 1983
National Assistance Act 1948
National Assistance (Amendment) Act 1951
National Health Service Act 1977
National Health Service and Community Care Act 1990
Nurses, Midwives and Health Visitors Act 1979
Nurses, Midwives and Health Visitors Act 1992
Offences Against the Person Act 1861
Prevention of Terrorism Act 1989
Public Health (Control of Diseases) Act 1984
Road Traffic Act 1976
Suicide Act 1961

1

Ethics, law and society

The subsequent chapters of this book will introduce you to ethical and legal issues relating to nursing practice. All nurses engaged in clinical practice will confront ethical dilemmas in the course of their career. Such dilemmas will take several different forms. A patient asks you if he has cancer. Do you tell him the truth? What if the consultant in charge of his care has instructed that the patient should not be told the true diagnosis because 'he could not cope'? A colleague is drinking heavily and her hands shake as she does a dressing. Do you blow the whistle on her? Some of the ethical questions which you will have to address are peculiar to nursing, but others may not be. Advances in medicine, particularly at the beginning and end of life, have generated new dilemmas of their own. Should artificial feeding be withdrawn from a patient in a persistent vegetative state? How do you respond when parents beg you not to treat their infant with severe hydrocephalus? Some commentators argue that these sort of dilemmas are concerned with medical not nursing practice, and nursing ethics should be separate from medical ethics, but that is not the approach we take. It may be that ultimately a doctor takes the final decision to discontinue treatment. However, today health care is multi-disciplinary and nurses will be members of a team caring for the patient. They should be informed of the issues and be centrally involved in decision-making in such cases. After all, if a patient is to be allowed to die it is the nurses who will care for him as he dies.

Nurses need to be involved in ethical debate for other reasons too. You will see that more and more emphasis is being put on the nurse's role as the patient's advocate. Advocates need to know what they are talking about. Crucial judgments must be made by society about the pace of developments in health care, about allocation of resources and the extent of patients' rights. The General Medical Council, the British Medical Association, the Royal College of Physicians and the other medical Royal Colleges play a public role in such debate, exercising great influence on government. Nursing bodies such as the Royal College of Nursing and the United Kingdom Central Council for Nursing, Midwifery and Health

Visiting are consulted too, and their voice should carry equal weight with the doctors. At local level, nurses should be fully represented on ethical committees. To participate fully in ethical debate the nurse must be adequately informed about the substance of that debate.

Nursing practice today

Nursing is in essence a dynamic process and current practice has advanced nursing far beyond its traditional boundaries. Nurses are no longer mere 'handmaidens'. Traditionally nurses played little part in making decisions about the care patients and clients received, but modern nursing practice places greater emphasis on the nurse's role in planning, implementing and evaluating nursing care. Any expansion of a nurse's role means greater responsibility and, as a consequence, increased accountability. Once a nurse exercises independent judgment she becomes answerable for the consequences of her decisions. She may be called to account by her peers, by her employers and ultimately by the courts.

Within what framework then do today's nurses practise their profession? Before answering that question we should perhaps acknowledge that there is still debate about whether or not nurses do constitute a profession. It is a debate beyond the scope of this work. For the lawyer-authors, at least, the answer is simple. Nurses are a clearly defined occupational group to whom Parliament has granted the privilege of self-regulation. Self-regulation, enjoyed by other groups such as lawyers and doctors, is seen as the hallmark of professional status. Self-regulation means that the profession itself defines the framework within which the professionals practise. So in the United Kingdom nursing practice is regulated by the United Kingdom Central Council for Nursing, Midwifery and Health Visiting, a grand title usually abbreviated to the UKCC.

Prior to 1979 nurses, midwives and health visitors each had their own separate regulatory system, but the Nurses, Midwives and Health Visitors Act 1979 brought the nursing professions together into one system ultimately controlled by the UKCC. The Council was entrusted with the mandate to 'establish and improve standards of training and professional conduct for Nurses, Midwives and Health Visitors'. Its functions include maintaining the register of nurses, midwives and health visitors, meeting European Community standards of training, advising on standards of professional conduct and disciplining nurses, midwives and health visitors charged with misconduct.

Under the 1979 Act the Council was composed of a maximum of forty-five members. The majority of Council members were nominated to the Council by the English, Welsh, Scottish and Northern Irish National Boards, whereas the majority of members of National Boards were elected by nurses themselves. But the Council was at best indirectly elected and there was no requirement that the National Boards should nominate elected members to the Council. The Nurses, Midwives and Health Visitors Act 1992 changed that position radically. The UKCC has increased its membership from forty-five to sixty and two-thirds of the members are directly elected by the profession itself.

This is not a book about the regulation of nursing so we do not elaborate on the organisation and powers of the UKCC. But its power and influence must not be underestimated. You cannot become a registered nurse unless the UKCC admits you to the register, and only the UKCC can end your career altogether. A hospital may dismiss you, patients may sue you, but if the UKCC finds you guilty of professional misconduct then you can be erased from the register and banned from practice altogether.

The UKCC is crucial in debates on ethical dilemmas in nursing, first, because Parliament has instructed it to advise on standards of practice and give ethical guidance to nurses and, second, because it is the body which can punish you for unethical conduct. The UKCC issues several documents advising on ethical standards of which the most important is the *Code of Professional Conduct for Nurses, Midwives and Health Visitors*. We discuss the detailed provisions of the Code throughout the book. However, as you will see, it does not comprise a simple list of 'do's and don'ts'. The Code directs you to the issues you must address in making judgments on ethical dilemmas; it does not tell you what to do in each and every case. You must, the Code demands, pay attention to ethics. So, what do we mean by ethics?

Ethics and morals

Ethics is a branch of philosophy concerned with the character and conduct of individuals, but this explanation may not be very meaningful until we answer another question – what is philosophy? People often make statements beginning with the phrase 'my philosophy on life is . . .'. This is usually followed with some detail about what they believe, what values they hold, and what judgments they make as a result of holding these beliefs and values. Most nurses are familiar with the term 'philosophy' from their involvement in developing ward and unit philosophies. A ward or unit philosophy usually consists of a series of statements on the beliefs held by the staff about individuals in general and how this influences the care they receive. So, for example, a ward philosophy may state that the nurses on ward fifty-three believe that each patient or client is a unique individual. The philosophy will then go on to detail the methods of care delivery which are utilised on ward fifty-three as a consequence of holding that belief.

Although this sense of philosophy is familiar, it does not fully describe what we shall be considering in this book. For this we will need to understand moral philosophy as it is defined as an academic subject. A useful explanation has been given by D. D. Raphael in his book *Moral Philosophy*. Raphael suggests that moral philosophy is the critical evaluation of beliefs and arguments. Moral philosophy in this sense is not just about statements made about the particular beliefs and values that individuals hold, but a critical evaluation of these beliefs and arguments. This in essence is what the term ethics means, the study of morality and moral issues. In other words, how do we evaluate actions and decide if they are right or wrong, good or bad?

The term 'ethical' has two rather different meanings. Firstly, it is used simply to relate to morality. Alternatively, it is also used to denote moral respectability or the moral soundness of an argument or a position. So, for example, to say that someone is acting ethically means that they are acting rightly, and to say that they are acting unethically means that they are acting wrongly from a moral perspective. The crucial issue is, however, not whether certain acts or judgments are ethical or unethical but *why* they are. We need to ask – is this practice, this custom, this course of action right or wrong?

If it is right or wrong, it will be so for a reason. Moral judgment presupposes the possibility of moral argument in which moral opinions are advanced supported by reason and, where appropriate, evidence. Where opinions are appropriately supported, they become 'judgments'.

Ethics not etiquette

In the context of health care practice, ethics inevitably relates to standards of behaviour. Ethical conduct is good conduct. Ethical practice is good practice. You must, however, be very careful to distinguish ethics from etiquette. Etiquette (or good manners) is a very elaborated, if not well articulated, normative system of rules. A normative system of rules attempts to establish standards of correct behaviour by the prescription of rules. The rules of good manners are very often rigidly enforced and there may be severe punishments for breaking such rules. However, the rules of etiquette are not necessarily moral rules and therefore not necessarily backed up by morality. For example, it is not unethical to eat with your fingers rather than with a knife and fork, although it may become so under certain contexts such as when in doing so you insult your host and hostess. Ethics and etiquette have often become confused in health care practice. For example, advice given to doctors on ethics up until relatively recently focused largely on injunctions not to speak ill of fellow doctors, not to try and 'poach' patients, and not to advertise. Aspiring barristers received 'ethical' advice on how to address judges and, again, not to denigrate their 'brothers'. Such advice had nothing to do with ethics but comprised a code of etiquette. Raanon Gillon used the phrase 'critical medical ethics' to describe the degree of reflection and critical evaluation demanded by true ethical discourse. 'Critical health care ethics' also allows people outside the profession to take part in that discourse. You might argue that nursing etiquette is none of the business of the three non-nurse authors of this work. Nursing ethics are the concern of us all.

So critical evaluation is central to ethics. With all normative systems except ethics it is always possible to say: 'OK, so these are the rules, but are they morally right and should I obey them?' The fact that they are the rules of good manners may constitute one reason for obeying them but that is not necessarily a moral reason. In the context of nursing practice, you will come across all sorts of rules and regulations, conventions and instructions given to you by people in authority. It is always a question for you as to whether you ought, morally speaking, to obey these regulations or instructions. You may be instructed by etiquette. Ethics demands you make judgments for yourself.

Ethics and culture

It is sometimes said that moralities are necessarily relative to a particular culture or society and that it is even a form of imperialism to suggest that the moral practices of another society, culture or even another period in history are unethical. To do so is to assert the superiority of our own society, culture or time over that of another and this alleged superiority can have no moral force. Moral relativism does not make sense and we will try to explain why.

If we believe something to be right or wrong it surely does not make sense to think that it can be right or wrong here and now, but not then and there. For example, if we believe that slavery is wrong, it makes no sense to say that it is wrong in Britain in the twentieth century but was perfectly acceptable in the southern states of America in the nineteenth century or in the Athens of Aristotle. To believe that it is wrong is to think there is something about it which makes it wrong, and as long as these features exist in these other societies then it will be wrong then and there as well. It would be odd indeed to say that murdering an innocent child is wrong in our society but perfectly acceptable and right in another society. So there seems to be something inconsistent about truly believing something to be right or wrong but believing it in such a half-hearted way that no criticism attaches to those who transgress as long as they do not live in our society or street or time. But there is another, larger problem with moral relativism.

If it is seriously claimed that we cannot criticise another culture, or another time or another society from outside, then it also cannot be criticised from inside. For whatever reasons a member of a particular society might have to find fault with the morality of that society, in so far as they hold good, these reasons would hold good if they were voiced outside as well. So, moral relativism implies the impossibility of moral progress since moral progress occurs when a society looks seriously at itself and finds fault. Take for example the progress of women's liberation in the United Kingdom. If, looking at our society 150 years ago, it was possible for members of that society to say that there were inadequate grounds for discriminating against women and treating them as second-class citizens, then the inadequacy of those grounds, in so far as that inadequacy was accessible to members of that society, would have been accessible to members of other societies. Whatever good reasons there are for the equal treatment of women with men, they are good whether they are voiced from within by a member of that society, or from without by external critics. The status of the criticism is the same in each case. We can accept moral relativism only if we are prepared to accept the impossibility of moral change.

Ethics and the law

So far we have said very little about the law, yet a central purpose of this book is to deal with both ethics and law. This is because ethical dilemmas very often provoke legal questions too. If you do not tell someone of a colleague's alcoholism and he injures a patient, might you be held liable in negligence? When a decision has to be made about withdrawing treatment so that a patient can die with dignity, should you seek the authority of the court? Might you and your colleagues risk prosecution for homicide? Law is crucial to nursing practice because of two key factors. Firstly, the law represents society's judgment on ethical standards. Legislation and judge-made law set the parameters of ethical conduct as perceived by society. You may not always think the law gets it right. Secondly, the law enforces sanctions against unethical behaviour both via imposition of criminal penalties and by imposing obligations on clients and patients. The UKCC can bar you from practice but the courts can send you to gaol.

However, do not overestimate the rule of law. Many nurses today are beginning to share doctors' fears about the intrusion of law into patient care. They fear an avalanche of litigation and 'ambulance-chasing' lawyers, but we shall try to demonstrate that such fears are exaggerated. Equally importantly, the law's usefulness in relation to ethical dilemmas is limited. The law is generally concerned to deter bad conduct and it plays little part in encouraging good conduct. You would be a poor nurse if you considered that ethical behaviour and good practice simply consisted in not falling foul of the law.

2

Nurses and ethics

An ethical dilemma occurs when there are at least two possible courses of action that may be taken but each option is problematic. All health professionals face ethical or moral dilemmas regularly in current clinical practice. The precise nature of the dilemmas may vary according to clinical details and so in some circumstances a dilemma may only be faced by doctors and in others, only faced by nurses. It would be unusual for only one type of health professional to care totally for a patient and so a multi-disciplinary approach to care is usually necessary. Because of this, health professionals will sometimes need to adopt a multi-disciplinary approach to solving ethical dilemmas as well. Listening to the opinions of others is often helpful to the person who ultimately has to make the decision. Health care by definition is a practical activity, and no matter how difficult or even impossible the ethical dilemmas may appear to be, a practical solution will usually have to be found. Reaching a solution involves moral reasoning and the application of ethical theory which is introduced in this chapter.

Ethical principles

People make moral judgments every day, usually without the need to refer to philosophers or ethical theories to assist them. Judgments of this sort are often based upon the behaviour believed to be acceptable or unacceptable in society. The beliefs that an individual may have about what constitutes morally acceptable behaviour will have been influenced in a variety of ways according to the culture to which the person belongs, their family, educational and recreational institutions and any religious beliefs that the person may have. There are certain rules in society to which people generally adhere, irrespective of their ethnic origin or religious beliefs. Examples of these rules are not killing an innocent human being, not telling lies, paying debts and keeping promises. Rules of this sort are taken seriously and anyone breaking them is likely to incur some

sort of penalty. The penalties are wide-ranging depending upon the severity of the case and whether as a result the person has also broken the law.
Someone who lies to a friend may lose that person's friendship, but someone who steals from a friend may both lose the friendship and face criminal proceedings.

Principles are fundamental moral rules that are used to justify actions
and behaviour. In everyday speech, people often refer to principles, for
example, when a person makes a statement like 'I acted on principle', or
'It is against my principles to tell lies.' What people are trying to do when
they speak in this way is to explain their actions by referring to a principle
or rule which they acknowledge governs their behaviour. So the person
who states that it is against her or his principles to tell lies, believes that
it is morally right to tell the truth and telling lies is therefore wrong.

A health professional faced with an ethical dilemma has to decide which
of the possible options is the right action to take and how choice of this
action over any others can be justified. Actions can then be explained by
demonstrating the ethical principles which justify them. The main ethical
principles applicable to nursing ethics are the principle of respect for persons,
respect for autonomy, justice, beneficence and non-maleficence. Application
of these principles will be explored in more detail in the following chapters.

Ethical theory

The origins of moral philosophy date from around 600 BC and from that
time to the present day, many ethical theories have been advanced. There
are, however, two schools of philosophical thought which have been particularly influential and which in many ways work in opposition to each
other. Theories of this sort can be collected under the broad headings of
consequentialism and deontology. We look firstly at consequentialism.

Consequentialism

One way of trying to decide if an action is the right thing to do or not is
to examine the consequences of performing that action. There are several
different versions of this type of ethical theory which can be put under the
general heading of consequentialism, but probably the most famous version of this approach is called utilitarianism.

1. Utilitarianism
This theory is generally associated with the writings of Jeremy Bentham
and John Stuart Mill, English philosophers who lived in the nineteenth
century. Mill was particularly interested in social and political reform and
was influenced by the writings of Jeremy Bentham, who suggested the

principle of utility as the foundation of morals. Mill attempted to refine some of Bentham's original statements without substantially changing the meaning of them. In *Utilitarianism*, Mill states the classical formulation of the principle of utility:

> The creed which accepts as the foundation of morals, Utility or the Greatest Happiness Principle, holds that actions are right in proportion as they tend to promote happiness, wrong as they tend to produce the reverse of happiness. By happiness is intended pleasure, and the absence of pain; by unhappiness, pain and the privation of pleasure.

What this means then is simply that an action can be thought of as morally correct if it brings about the greatest amount of happiness and prevents pain.

Suppose that you visit your elderly uncle who is seriously ill and not expected to live very long. Towards the end of your visit, your uncle gives you £500 which he says he has been saving to give to the Royal Society for the Protection of Birds. Your uncle asks you to make sure that the society receives the money as he is now incapable of doing so himself. Later that evening you watch a programme about the work of Oxfam in areas of East Africa experiencing drought and famine, and you come to the conclusion that your uncle's £500 would be better spent by giving it to Oxfam rather than the RSPB. You feel that saving human lives is more important than saving birds and so decide to donate the money to Oxfam without your uncle's knowledge. When you next visit your uncle, you tell him that you have sent the money to the RSPB as he requested.

Lying to a dying man or failing to carry out a simple request he has made may appear to be a callous act, but an apparent justification is open to you by appealing to the principle of utility. In general, being deceitful is not considered morally acceptable, but in these circumstances you are attempting to make a contribution to relieve the suffering of starving people. You could argue that in sending money to Oxfam, you are promoting the happiness of starving people. In the same way, by lying to your uncle you are also promoting his happiness, as you know he would be upset if you told him the truth. The RSPB, however, may not agree with you. The society may feel that its interests are being harmed by being deprived of the £500. You could argue that it is not that you disapprove of helping birds, but that you consider saving human lives to have more importance. Overall it has to be decided whether saving human lives is of more importance than saving birds. To justify lying in these circumstances does not mean that you place no value on honesty or that there may not be other circumstances when it will not be possible morally to justify lying to someone within a utilitarian framework.

This example shows that actions can be judged to be right or wrong depending on their consequences and the amount of happiness that can be derived for all people concerned. The aim is to produce the greatest amount of happiness for the greatest number of people. There are difficulties with this sort of approach and one of the main criticisms that has been made of utilitarianism is that there are other things to take into consideration as well as happiness, things like virtue, love, knowledge or truth. Questions have also been raised as to how the amount of happiness to be generated by actions can be accurately assessed. Another difficulty with utilitarianism is the emphasis that it places on promoting happiness for the greatest number, and it is possible to justify circumstances that would usually be thought of as unjust. The members of a community may, for example, believe that the greatest amount of happiness could be generated for them by expelling members of an ethnic minority who live within the area. In order to persuade these people to move elsewhere, life is made intolerable for them so that they are forced to leave the area, thereby promoting the greatest amount of good for the greatest amount of people, that is, the indigenous community.

2. Classical utilitarianism

Despite these difficulties, utilitarianism has maintained its popularity as an ethical theory although it has been modified by other writers in an attempt to overcome the obvious criticisms of the theory. Bentham and Mill have therefore become known as classical or hedonistic utilitarians (from the Greek *hedone*, meaning pleasure) because their version of the theory defines happiness as the only good end. Other utilitarians are described as pluralists as they take into consideration other things besides happiness such as virtue, truth or love. Other types of utilitarianism make a distinction between what is termed act utilitarianism and rule utilitarianism.

3. Act and rule utilitarianism

Act utilitarians believe that each individual action should be considered according to the consequences that are produced, whereas rule utilitarians believe that there are general rules which determine whether acts are right or wrong, such as 'Do not kill' or 'Do not steal'. In the example above, an attempt was made to justify telling lies to a dying man by appealing to the principle of utility. This sort of justification works for some forms of utilitarianism, but is an embarrassment to rule utilitarians. It was to overcome these sorts of difficulties that rule utilitarianism was devised. An act utilitarian, if unsure whether he or she should tell a lie, would consider the action of telling the lie in this particular circumstance and then assess the consequences of telling the lie. The act utilitarian would then decide if in telling the lie he or she would promote the greatest amount of good.

In contrast, a rule utilitarian would believe in the general rule that you should speak the truth and so would not consider the consequences of this particular action in isolation. The rule utilitarian is already committed to the belief that the greatest amount of good can be obtained overall if people tell the truth and the situations thus have to be considered on an individual basis. The rule utilitarian would therefore reach a different conclusion about telling lies to the dying man in the example described above. The rule utilitarian would not be able to justify sending the money to Oxfam rather than the RSPB, even though he or she may also think that it is a more worthy cause. The rule utilitarian will be committed to a belief in a general rule about speaking the truth, and so would either have to comply with the uncle's request, or send the money to Oxfam, but tell him that he or she has done so.

4. Preference utilitarianism

So far the types of utilitarianism discussed all rely on an understanding of values, such as happiness, which are common to all people. Some utilitarians believe that there are other things of comparable moral worth such as knowledge or love, and what an individual wants is also of moral importance. Another form of utilitarianism, preference utilitarianism, attempts to overcome these difficulties.

Preference utilitarianism relies on promoting or maximising the preferences that separate individuals have in order to judge if something is morally right or not. This allows a person's own particular desires and not just a general term such as happiness to be taken into account. For example, a dying person in great pain might prefer to be given a lethal injection (if this was allowed by the law), so that he could be allowed to die and end his suffering. However, another dying person in great pain might prefer to live for as long as possible even though she was suffering.

While all types of utilitarianism are consequentialist theories, not all types of consequentialism are utilitarian theories. Because of the different types of utilitarian theory that have developed, it is easier to gather them all under the general term of consequentialism. This term describes the main point upon which all the differing versions agree, which is that the consequences of actions determine if an act is morally right or wrong.

Deontology

Deontology, the other major ethical theory, is in complete contrast to consequentialism. The deontologist (from the Greek word *deon* meaning duty) believes that duty is the foundation of morality and that an act can be judged as either morally right or wrong in itself irrespective of the consequences that are produced. Actions, therefore, such as telling the truth and keeping promises are thought of as good in themselves and should always be promoted. The first question that this theory raises is 'How can you know that certain actions are good in themselves?' One of the justifications for this approach can be found in the writings of the Old and New Testaments of the Bible and those with religious beliefs believe that these are the rules or laws commanded by God. Those without religious beliefs either explain this knowledge through human intuition and common sense or argue that natural laws and rights exist which can be shown by human reasoning.

1. Religious justification

All of the major world religions are founded upon a belief that a God (or Gods) is responsible for the creation of the world and all that is in it, including human beings. God has provided his people with moral laws that are to be obeyed and in the Christian tradition at least it is necessary to obey these moral laws in order to secure a place in Heaven in the life after death. An example of these sorts of laws can be seen in the Ten Commandments. However, as religions and denominations within religions have developed, extra moral laws are often added that are not specified within the basic texts, as for example those that are an essential part of the Roman Catholic faith.

This implies that individuals are not capable of acting morally without the existence of a God who can show people the right and wrong way to act. Bertrand Russell, an English philosopher of this century, did not think that a belief in God gave a sufficient justification for morally correct behaviour. Russell's suggestion is that if someone is sure that there is a difference between right and wrong, that person will need to recognise that what God commands is good or right. If they are capable of doing this, then they recognise that right and wrong have a meaning independent of God's will. The idea that God himself must recognise the difference between right and wrong, even if he has created the difference, claims that he commands particular things because they are good rather than that they are good because he commands them. If what God commands is good, it is so because right and wrong have a meaning independent of God's will. God himself must be able to recognise the difference between right and wrong and order his commands accordingly. If this is so, right and wrong exist independently of God.

According to this view, it is not an accident that, for example, the Ten Commandments take the form that they do. God chose those particular Commandments because they were the right ones to choose. The alternative view, that whatever God had commanded would have been good for that reason, would have left it theoretically possible for God to have commanded slaughtering the innocent. If this is inconceivable, it is so not because we believe that whatever God commands is for that reason good, but rather that we believe God chooses good commands. If this reasoning is correct, then it is difficult to explain why someone should rely on God as the only being that can recognise the difference between right and wrong. There are also difficulties in understanding where the meaning of right and wrong came from if not directly from God and who or what was responsible for their existence.

If a belief in God is necessary for people to recognise the differences between right and wrong, then it follows that people who do not hold this belief should have lower moral standards than those who do hold religious beliefs. Examples from history and from the present day do not, however, appear to support this; for example, many wars have been waged based on a religious justification. Another difficulty with a religious justification for the basis of moral rules is that not only are there inconsistencies about what constitutes these moral laws between religious groups, but many people do not have a religious faith of any sort whatsoever. Because of this it would be impossible to suggest that a religious justification for the existence of moral rules could be used as a basis of morality for people other than believers. This is not to say that people who profess religious beliefs cannot explain their own moral code by the existence of God, but it does not establish that non-believers can be obliged to live their lives according to such a moral code.

2. Kantian ethics

One of the main contributors to deontological ethical theories was Immanuel Kant, a German philosopher in the eighteenth century. Unlike Bentham and Mill, whose ethical theories had a practical dimension in social and political reform, Kant was a professor of logic and metaphysics without any sort of public life. For Kant, the foundation of morality lay in what he called the categorical imperative which is formulated in his book *Groundwork of the Metaphysic of Morals*, translated by Paton as *The Moral Law*. A categorical imperative is a moral command and Kant's version states that firstly, individuals should act in a way that could be made a law for everyone else and secondly, they should treat human beings as ends in themselves, not just means to an end. For Kant, then, whether an action is morally right or wrong depends entirely on following moral rules such as telling the truth, being honest or keeping promises.

The example of deceiving your dying uncle used to illustrate utilitarianism earlier in this chapter has a different conclusion if viewed from a Kantian perspective. By telling your uncle a lie, you are breaking one of the accepted moral rules. Although you feel that in doing so you are taking the best course of action by saving starving human beings and protecting your uncle from distress, the categorical imperative does not allow any exceptions to the rule. If you accept this type of rule, it has to hold in every circumstance without exception, whatever the consequences of the action. This is the important difference between this type of theory and any form of consequentialism. Consequentialist theories judge the moral worth of an action by the consequences of that action, but deontological theories judge the moral worth of an action by the action itself, irrespective of the consequences.

Deontological theories tend to emphasise obligations. They concentrate on the particular actions that we are obliged to perform rather than on the consequences which we ought to bring about. For this reason, we need to say a little here about the nature of obligation.

Obligation

Obligation can be described as what we ought to do, or how we ought to act, in a given situation. By using this term, two assumptions are made. The first is that you can actually perform the action. For example, I may be persuaded that I ought to scale the north face of the Eiger because I would appreciate the view from the top, but as I have no knowledge of mountain climbing I would be unable to do so. This is sometimes encapsulated in the saying ' "Ought" implies "can" '. To say that someone ought to do something implies that they can actually do it. The second assumption is that the person has a choice about whether to perform the action or not. Suppose that I see a blind person having difficulty crossing a busy road; I may feel that I ought to go and help that person. Clearly this is an action I am able to perform, but I also have a choice. I could help the blind person across the road or I could simply ignore the fact that he or she is in difficulty and continue with whatever I was doing. An obligation to perform an act is therefore that which will morally compel me to assist the blind person crossing the road rather than ignoring her or him.

It is important to be aware that there are different sorts of obligations that people can have. For example, we talk about contractual obligations, family obligations and moral obligations. Where individuals agree to do certain things, they make in a sense a 'contract', whether this is formally written down and spelled out or simply an informal agreement. The obligations that people have flow from the agreement they have made. Family obligations differ in character because we say that people have certain obligations simply by virtue of the fact that they are related to one another or they live in a family situation, whether or not they are genetically related to one another. So, for example, we say that someone who is a mother, whether genetically or because of the role that she has assumed, has an obligation to look after her child. She has this obligation by virtue of the role that she plays or the relationship in which she stands. We use the term moral obligation to refer to those obligations whether contractual, family or of any other kind that we feel ought to be both felt and discharged.

Health professionals have obligations of all sorts. They have obligations which are contractual in nature because they have agreed to the terms and conditions of their employment as a health professional. They have role obligations similar to those which family members acquire in respect of one another. Where someone takes on the role of a carer they create for themselves obligations that they would not have had, had they not assumed that role. Equally, health professionals have moral obligations of many sorts. For example, they have an obligation to respect a patient's confidences, to have respect for a patient's autonomy, to do good (the principle of beneficence), and also to do no harm (the principle of non-maleficence). There are, however, situations when conflict occurs between differing sorts of obligations. Suppose that a patient tells a nurse that he has undergone some surgery in the past that he has not informed anyone else in the hospital about. The nurse is aware that the information is relevant to the treatment that the patient is currently undergoing, but the patient asks the nurse to respect his confidence. The nurse may feel that she has an obligation to the patient not to pass on the information that has been given to her, but she also has an obligation not to harm the patient. If a nurse fails to give other members of the health care team the relevant information, the patient may be harmed as a result.

J. Harris in *The Value of Life* has argued that health professionals do not have any special obligations at all, but are subject to the same sort of duties as any other person in society. All individuals have a duty to respect confidences or do no harm because of their respect for other people, and this is not just the duty of health professionals. While this is a plausible argument, the UKCC identifies certain obligations as part of the professional role, and this will be expanded upon in the chapters on confidentiality, autonomy, responsibility and accountability.

Rights

As well as recognising certain obligations that health professionals are under when caring for patients, another perspective on this can be shown by describing the rights that people have or claim to have. These may include a right to life, a right to a hospital bed, a right to a vote or a right to freedom of speech. The terms 'rights' and 'rights-based theories' are popular in many different sections of society, health care being only one of them. The Patient's Charter, for example, which became effective from April 1992, sets out ten rights which every citizen can claim under the National Health Service. These include a right to health care based on need, a right to admission for treatment within two years of being placed on a waiting list and a right to access of manually held records from November 1991. In addition, the Charter also specifies nine standards of care that should be achieved by those involved in the management and delivery of health care. To say that a person has a right to something means that person is able to make a claim upon some other person or an institution. It is important that the person can justify this claim by using principles and rules which may be either legal or moral.

Certain rights are recognised as legal rights because they are protected by law and the law can therefore be used to justify a claim to such rights. In a similar way, moral rights are claims that can be justified using moral principles. Some people would argue that, irrespective of what the law says about the permissibility of abortion, every foetus has a right to life and should not be aborted under any circumstances. Someone arguing in this way could appeal to a natural right to life that all individuals can claim.

Natural rights

Some people believe in the existence of what are termed 'natural rights' which are absolute rights that individuals can claim. Rights of this sort were called natural because they were derived from the concept of natural law which has its origins in ancient Greece and was an important part of the philosophy of the Stoics in particular. The Stoics believed that there was a natural order to everything that occurred in the natural world such as the movements of planets or changes in the seasons. Nothing happened by chance, as everything and everybody in the world had a purpose which was designed by God. Stoicism was not confined to Greece and many of the later Stoic philosophers were Roman, and it was the Roman lawyers who first applied the principles of natural law and natural justice. At first Roman law, the *jus civile* (civil law), only applied to Roman citizens, leaving foreigners with no protection under the law and therefore no rights. Later another type of law, the *jus gentium* (international law), was developed and applied to all people, citizens and non-citizens alike. People were then able to defend their rights by appealing to the principles of natural justice.

By recognising natural justice in this way, it was an inevitable consequence that natural rights which people could claim would also be recognised. Natural rights may still be explained as being God's commands by some people, but it is not always necessary for natural rights to be justified in this way. More commonly the term human rights is now used and this relates to rights that exist as a result of the way that people live as part of society. The Universal Declaration of Human Rights produced by the General Assembly of the United Nations in 1948 is an example of this. The document contains thirty articles detailing the rights that individuals can claim, such as a right to life, liberty, security of person, equality before the law, nationality and free basic education. Some countries, like the United States and France, also identify in the country's constitution certain rights that their citizens have.

To claim a right to something involves the claim that others are to respect that right. For example, someone may claim that they have a right to life and in doing so they are claiming that others have an obligation not to kill them and so violate that right. Claiming a right to life and making others obliged not to kill raises some difficult questions. In ordinary circumstances a right to life should not be violated, but there are situations when this right is not always thought of as absolute. In times of war, members of the armed services, as well as civilians, are deprived of their right to life. The armed services of the opposing side do not have an obligation to respect that right. If anything, they have an obligation to violate that right in respect of service personnel. Another example when the right to life is not considered absolute is if a person kills another in self-defence. Clearly there are arguments that can justify killing in these circumstances (although pacifists would probably not agree in the former case), so it does not make sense to say that any right claimed is absolute and places others under an obligation not to violate that right at any time.

The difficulty lies in justifying when rights may either be violated or overridden when they conflict with other rights. There are many debates that centre on people claiming rights that are in conflict with their opponents. For example, some people claim the right to be free to smoke cigarettes in public places, while others claim a right to be in a smoke-free environment. Supporters of abortion may claim that a woman has a right to choose what she does to her own body, while opponents may claim that the foetus has a right to life. In these examples, and in all other situations when people claim rights that conflict, it has to be decided which right has the strongest claim and so may override other rights. Where conflicting rights are claimed, it may be impossible to reconcile them.

This brief survey of two main types of ethical theory and the sorts of concepts used by these theories, such as rights, obligations, duties and so on, has, we hope, given you a general sense of how moral arguments might proceed and how moral dilemmas of the sort that arise in health care can be addressed. Much confusion, we are sure, will be left in your mind at this point. Our intention is that the confusion will, to a certain extent, be resolved as we look more specifically at particular issues as our discussion advances. It is our hope that by the end of the book you will have a good sense of how particular dilemmas in health care are addressed in terms of the theories, principles and concepts we have briefly surveyed at the start.

3

Nurses and the law

Some knowledge and understanding of the law has become a vital part of nursing education today for at least two reasons. First, many people argue that any educated person should be familiar with the principles that govern our behaviour and relationships with each other. Citizens need to know their rights and obligations. Second, as a nurse you take on particular responsibilities which make you more susceptible to the scrutiny of the law than the average individual. These responsibilities arise because as a nursing professional you offer unique skills and by providing nursing services you accept responsibility for those under your care and for your actions. It is therefore essential that you are aware of the situations in which those professional skills create legal obligations so that you may act accordingly.

The expanding scope of nursing practice has heightened professional interest in the relationship between law and nursing because some nurses feel that increased responsibility and independence will involve more onerous legal liabilities. This remains to be seen. What every nurse should be familiar with is a general outline of the legal system, so that she has a proper appreciation of the role that the law will play in her future career.

In this chapter those areas of law which are most relevant to nursing will be explained, and they include the following:

1. Criminal law
2. Civil law

Criminal law

Criminal law concerns the kind of conduct by any individual which will be punished by the State. The behaviour in question is thought to be so damaging to society as a whole that it warrants intervention and punishment by the State. To be convicted of a crime the prosecution must have proved that a prohibited act was committed (*actus reus*) and a guilty mind (*mens rea*) was present. Translated into plain English this means that a person must have intended to commit the crime, or was reckless or negligent in doing the criminal act. Obvious examples of crimes are murder, manslaughter, theft, rape and illegal abortion. Prosecutions are pursued under the name of the Crown. A person accused of a crime is arrested and charged by the police and then the Crown Prosecution Service decides whether or not to prosecute. Only the most serious crimes result in imprisonment, and are tried by a Crown Court judge in wig and gown, together with a jury. Minor matters are dealt with in local Magistrates' Courts.

Criminal law is not usually concerned with negligent acts unless death is caused: for example, when a grossly negligent overdose kills a patient. In such a case a nurse could be charged with manslaughter. Usually a mistake made in the course of a nurse's duties will not be punished under criminal law.

Civil law

Civil law is concerned with the relationships between individuals. Aggrieved individuals, and not the State, initiate proceedings against the wrongdoer. The outcome of these proceedings will usually be an award of compensation (damages) or an order (injunction) to stop acting unlawfully. The law which governs these relationships is extensive and has to be sub-divided into several further sub-categories. Those categories most relevant to nursing are described in the following paragraphs.

Tort

Tort means 'wrong' in French, and in England the law of tort is very much concerned with wrongs. Certain sorts of behaviour are prohibited by tort even though not punished as crimes. The law provides that individuals owe each other obligations because they live together in society and the law of tort enforces those obligations and protects the rights which flow from them.

There are certain clearly recognised torts, but the list is not definitive and new torts have developed over time. For example, the courts are currently developing a tort of harassment. Examples of established torts include negligence, assault and battery, and libel. So if, for example, you are found to have been negligent in administering an overdose, the patient (as plaintiff) might be able to sue you (as defendant) in an action for negligence to obtain compensation.

Contract law

Contract law is concerned with agreements or promises which individuals make or arrange between themselves. In England agreements are only legally enforceable if both parties have received something of value in return for their promise or obligation to each other. Mere promises are not enforced as such. Contract law is really only relevant to private health care practice, and to the nurse as an employee. NHS patients, because they do not pay the nurse or the hospital for their care directly, have no contract either with the nurse or the NHS authorities. Contrary to popular belief, a contract need not be written. A legally enforceable contract is any agreement for value which has been made with an intention to have legal consequences and can be made, not only in writing, but orally, or may even be implied by the conduct of the parties. If you are paid to provide private care for an elderly patient at home, you have a contract regardless of the fact nothing is ever written down.

Not every document, even if it is called a contract, is in fact a legal contract. The new NHS 'contracts' which were created under the National Health Service and Community Care Act 1990 provide an example; the ordinary law of contract is expressly made inapplicable under the Act. The Department of Health, not the courts, interprets and enforces these 'pseudo-contracts'.

Family law

Family law encompasses the law relating to marriage, divorce and child care. It is especially important in health care in terms of professional and parental responsibilities to children and is probably most relevant in the areas of health visiting and emergency operations on babies and children. Note that parental rights to control the treatment of their children are not unlimited.

Administrative law

The law which governs the powers and duties of public authorities is known as administrative law. Health authorities and hospital trusts are regulated by administrative law through the power of the courts to review their decisions and policies. By these means (an action for judicial review) individuals can assert their rights and challenge public authority decision-making. Patients and nurses alike can question, for example, selection criteria or health authority policy. The court then rules on the legality of the policy.

How laws are made

You may think that all laws are made by Parliament in the form of Acts of Parliament (statutes) such as the Abortion Act 1967. In fact a great deal of the law is still made by the judges who adjudicate on particular cases and give a judgment which then forms a precedent in subsequent court cases. Judge-made law is often referred to as the 'common law' to distinguish it from statute-law made by Parliament. Confusingly though, common law is also sometimes used in two quite different senses. First, common law is used to refer to the basic nature of English law, which is so heavily based on judge-made law, to distinguish it from the civil law of Continental Europe, which is based on very detailed Codes of Law derived from the Napoleonic Code. Second, common law is sometimes the term used to describe areas of law concerned with relations between individuals (such as tort and contract) as opposed to public law, i.e. the laws governing the relationship of the State and its subjects (such as criminal law and administrative law).

However, important though the judge-made common law is, Parliament has supreme power. Legislation enacted by Parliament can change any judge-made rules. We have no written constitution in the United Kingdom so, subject to our membership of the European Community, Parliament can enact whatever laws it likes. Imagine that in both the United Kingdom and the United States of America the legislature sought to pass a law banning abortion under any circumstances, even if the mother faces death. Women in the USA could challenge such a law as unconstitutional, violating their right to life and privacy. No such remedy exists in this country directly although cases of this sort can be taken to the European Court of Human Rights.

Although a great deal of the law governing your legal obligations as a nurse is judge-made, laws determining the structure of our health service are made by Parliament. And of course, as we saw in Chapter One, provision for the regulation of nursing is made by statute in the Nurses, Midwives and Health Visitors Acts of 1979 and 1992. Highly controversial issues such as access to and control of fertility treatment will generally result in legislation, for example, the Human Fertilisation and Embryology Act 1990. You need to know something of how legislation is made because, when legislation affects nurses, you ought to have a voice in the process and understand when and how to lobby Parliament to get your view across. Doctors are very good at pressing their opinions on MPs.

All legislation must be approved by both Houses of Parliament, i.e. the elected House of Commons and the unelected House of Lords. The majority of Acts are initiated by the government of the day and a few are introduced by individual members of Parliament, for example the Abortion Act 1967 which was introduced by David Steel MP. Although approval of both Houses is needed, the House of Lords can usually only delay legislation (up to a year) and not veto it altogether.

To understand how legislation is enacted, and how you as a nurse can influence the process, three sorts of legislation will be looked at as follows:

1. Party political legislation
2. Non-party political, social or moral issues legislation
3. Private Members' Bills

1. Party political legislation

An example of such legislation is the National Health Service and Community Care Act 1990. A political party, in this case the Conservative Party, develops a policy on health care, incorporates it in its election manifesto on which it wins a general election, and forms a government.

Once in power, Department of Health civil servants examine the policy; the Treasury costs the policy; and Cabinet Ministers consider the civil servants' advice. Outside experts (e.g. the Royal College of Nursing) are consulted and a Green Paper (preliminary proposal) may be published. The Green Paper is debated and further experts may be consulted. Their opinions will be evaluated, but if the Government is determined to push the policy through they will issue a White Paper (final proposal) followed by a Bill which sets out the proposals in legislative form.

The Bill is presented to Parliament, usually going to the Commons first where it receives a formal and unopposed First Reading. The press and the public comment on the Bill, which is then presented for its Second Reading when the principles of the legislation are debated in the House. The Opposition divides the House by calling for a vote. In such legislation MPs have no choice in voting. A 'three line whip' is issued ordering them to follow the Party line. So the Government rarely loses. A Parliamentary committee studies the Bill in detail and reports back to the House with suggested amendments. This is known as the Report Stage. Details that do not affect major principles in the Bill may get changed.

The Bill then has its Third Reading and if passed, as it will be, it goes to the Lords where the process is repeated but where there is more likely to be a Government defeat on detail. Expert opinion carries more weight in the Lords. If the House of Lords changes the Bill it has to go back to the Commons before receiving the Royal Assent from the monarch, who never says no! The legislation is then a complete Act of Parliament (statute). As is obvious, lobbying in this sort of case may result in minor concessions, but is unlikely to overturn the whole thrust of proposed government action.

2. Non-party political, social or moral issues legislation

A good example of such legislation is the Human Fertilisation and Embryology Act 1990. In this sort of case the government may set up a committee of enquiry like the Warnock committee on embryology. The committee asks all those concerned to submit evidence to it and finally reports back to the Government with proposals. Further discussion papers may be issued and ultimately a White Paper is published. A Bill is introduced into Parliament often starting in the Lords, and the procedure is then as in 1. above. The potential to influence the nature of statutes in this sort of case is much greater. Doctors involved in *in vitro fertilisation* lobbied very successfully to ensure that embryo research remained lawful.

3. Private Members' Bills

These are Bills introduced by individual backbenchers. A ballot is held among backbenchers for the opportunity to introduce a Bill of his or her choice, and the first four or five in the ballot are usually made law. Debates take place on Friday afternoons and controversial Bills may be talked out so that no time is left for their introduction. Exceptionally the Government may give a Private Member's Bill extra time, as with the 1967 Abortion Act, because they sympathise with the Bill but do not want to endorse it officially.

The limits of primary legislation

No Act of Parliament can lay down in detail all the rules and procedures needed to implement new policies and proposals. The Act may therefore empower relevant Departments to make regulations (Statutory Instruments) and these regulations implement the Act. Acts of Parliament are often referred to as *primary legislation* and statutory instruments as *secondary legislation*. The Nurses, Midwives and Health Visitors Acts 1979 and 1992, as primary legislation, contain little specific detail but empower the UKCC to make Statutory Instruments which are legally binding for those to whom they apply.

Statutory interpretation

It is virtually impossible for even primary and secondary legislation together to cover every possible eventuality. In practice, a statute may be found to be unclear on certain issues, and judges must then interpret the legislation. The case of *Royal College of Nursing* v. *DHSS* (1981) illustrates this. The Abortion Act 1967 stipulated that in order for an abortion to be lawful the termination of pregnancy had to be performed by a registered medical practitioner. The RCN became concerned that where an abortion was performed by prostaglandin induction, nurses left in charge of the procedure were in effect performing the operation, and thereby acting illegally. When the Act was passed in 1967 abortions were only carried out via surgery. The House of Lords interpreted the Act so that nurses who carry out terminations by induction are entitled to the protection afforded by the Act and thereby would not be acting criminally.

Department of Health guidance

The Department of Health frequently gives formal guidance to health authorities and practitioners on legal and ethical issues relating to practice. The advice may often deal with doubtful legal questions, for example, the circular on contraceptive advice to be given to girls under sixteen. The Department's view of the law was challenged in *Gillick* v. *West Norfolk and Wisbech AHA* (1985). DoH guidance can be crucial in medical litigation if a doctor or nurse is sued for malpractice. Failure to comply with the Department's advice on safety procedures may be difficult to justify. Formal advice from professional bodies such as the UKCC will also be taken very seriously in any court proceeding.

How judge-made law is made

We noted earlier that much of the law relating to a nurse's professional practice and patients' rights has evolved from judge-made law, not from any sort of legislation, i.e. the common law. Common law depends on the system of precedent. Precedents are simply decisions on earlier similar disputes which bind future judgments. To work, the system depends on a hierarchy of the courts because judgments made by higher courts bind all lower courts. Thus you need to know something about the court system (see Figure 1).

The House of Lords

The most senior judges in the country, the Law Lords, are those who sit in the House of Lords. In legal cases before the House of Lords only these specially appointed Law Lords can participate in hearings. Ordinary dukes, earls and barons, etc., are not allowed to take part! A ruling by the House of Lords (comprising five Law Lords), like that in Mrs Gillick's case, binds all lower courts. A later hearing in the House of Lords very rarely results in the House of Lords itself changing its mind.

The Court of Appeal

The Court of Appeal is just one rung lower than the House of Lords in the hierarchy and is therefore bound by all judgments of the House of Lords and earlier judgments of its own. Three Lord Justices sit together to hear important cases. Court of Appeal decisions bind all lower courts.

The High Court

The High Court is where most cases raising important questions of principle begin. High Court judges, whether sitting alone or in a two/three-man

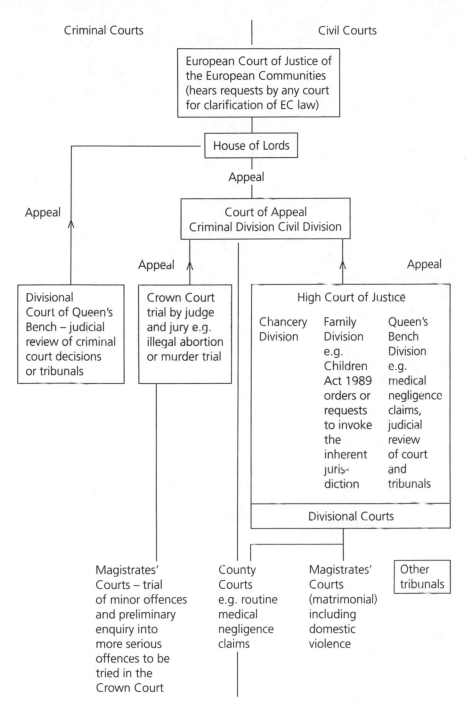

Figure 1   The Court hierarchy

court, are bound by all House of Lords and Court of Appeal judgments. High Court judgments are merely persuasive for other High Court judges but bind all lower courts.

In effect, all law making is done in these higher echelons of the judicial hierarchy. County and Crown Court judges and magistrates largely apply the law and adjudicate on disputes about facts.

Precedent – how does it work?

It is all very well knowing which set of judges make the precedents, but how on earth does the system work? In any case the judge will apply any relevant law that already exists. What the judge actually pronounces as the result of the case and the reason for his decision is known as the *ratio decidendi*. It is this ruling that sets the precedent. In the course of the judgment the judge may also make other comments and statements of opinion. These *obiter dicta* (other things that are said) are not binding on future courts but may influence later decisions.

To illustrate the process, first consider whether a woman with severe learning disabilities can ever be sterilised without her consent. Most countries have statutes governing if and when non-consensual sterilisation is lawful, but no British Act of Parliament addresses the question. So how can you work out what the law requires? We start with a basic common law principle that any physical contact with another person normally constitutes a battery (assault) unless the person has expressly or implicitly consented to that contact (see Chapter Four). When a child is too young to give her or his own consent, parents may authorise any treatment which is in her or his best interests. But parental authority ceases when the child reaches eighteen and there is no provision for any proxy consent for adults. So how can you lawfully treat an adult woman incapable of consenting on her own behalf? If a patient cannot consent to sterilisation and no one else may consent on her behalf, will a battery be committed where the patient is treated? The following cases illustrate how precedent developed an answer.

In 1976 the case of *Re D* was decided in the High Court. Mrs Justice Heilbron forbade the sterilisation of an eleven-year-old girl (D) who suffered from Soto's Syndrome and whose mother wanted her to be sterilised. Even though the mother's consent had been given, the court had to consider whether the treatment was in D's best interests. The judge decided that at eighteen D might be capable of deciding for herself and, therefore, immediate sterilisation was not in her best interests. *Re D* appeared to suggest non-consensual sterilisation would not be lawful in England.

Re B followed in 1987. B was a girl of seventeen with a mental age of six and very limited communication skills, and her behaviour was described as 'sexually provocative'. Again, the question was really whether or not such treatment was in B's best interests. The High Court decision in *Re D* could not bind the House of Lords. The Lords identified a number of factual matters which differentiated this case from *Re D*. Most importantly B was much nearer adulthood and it was unlikely that she would ever be able to decide and give consent on her own. In this situation the House of Lords decided that, in the last resort, a girl under eighteen could lawfully be sterilised where her interests required such surgery and the court agreed with her parents that this was the best course of action.

The House of Lords' decision in *Re B* was then considered in *T* v. *T* (1988). T was nineteen and more severely disabled than B. She became pregnant and her mother and doctors thought that the pregnancy should be terminated and T sterilised. As T was not a child, no one could legally give a proxy consent for her but at the same time she was incapable of giving a meaningful consent. The doctors went to court for a declaration (a statement of the law) as to whether such treatment would be lawful despite the absence of consent. No case law existed on this particular point and so the court could only refer to cases decided on non-consensual treatment of disabled children. Mr Justice Wood, in the High Court, held that where a patient would never be capable of consenting to proposed treatment on her own behalf it would be lawful to carry out treatment in her interests where good medical practice 'demands' that such treatment be performed.

Finally the issue came before the House of Lords in *F* v. *Berkshire Health Authority* (1989). F was a thirty-five-year-old patient with learning disabilities living in a hospital. She had formed a sexual relationship with a male patient and the hospital sought to have her sterilised. Their Lordships upheld the High Court decision and confirmed that a patient incapable of consenting on her own behalf may lawfully be sterilised, and set out conditions which must be met by doctors seeking to do so (see Chapter Ten).

From these cases you can see how precedent is used to develop law in new areas. *Re D* demonstrated an attitude wary of sterilising children with learning disabilities; this was slowly developed into a more permissive attitude which allows the sterilisation of adults with learning disabilities if it is considered to be in their best interests.

Nurses in court

Law-making is very much the preserve of the higher courts, and a nurse's actual experience of court proceedings is likely to be at a lower level. A nurse may have to appear as a witness when a patient sues for medical negligence, she may herself be sued or be a party to proceedings to protect a child or other vulnerable patient, or she might go to court to challenge decisions of her managers or health authority or employers. Let us look briefly at the different sorts of courts you as a nurse may come in contact with professionally.

1. Magistrates' Courts

Magistrates deal mainly with minor criminal offences and preliminary hearings relating to more serious charges. In the second situation the magistrates commit the accused for trial at the Crown Court. A nurse accused of a crime in her professional capacity will probably be appearing in a case of the second kind and would be tried in the Crown Court by a judge and jury. But as a witness she might have to go to the Magistrates' Court in a domestic case involving testifying to injuries involving a battered wife.

2. Crown Courts

A judge and a jury try serious criminal offences. If a nurse's evidence is required she may be subpoenaed, i.e. her attendance in court is demanded and as a witness she is obliged by law to answer all questions. Examples of cases in which you might be involved are criminal abortions or murder (euthanasia). As a witness you cannot claim any sort of privilege to entitle you to refuse to give evidence. If you are the accused, you are not obliged to give evidence, but if you do you must answer all questions. This right to silence is currently under review by the Government.

3. County Court

In the County Court a local judge hears civil disputes such as medical negligence claims which do not exceed £50,000. In family proceedings and child care cases only certain nominated local judges may adjudicate.

4. The High Court (Queen's Bench Division)

This is the likely venue for an action for medical negligence where either the claim is for more than £50,000 compensation or it involves any complicated legal question. The nurse may be the defendant or, much more likely, a vital witness in an action brought against a medical practitioner and the health authority.

The Queen's Bench Division also hears challenges to the legality of decisions of public authorities including health authorities and regulatory bodies like the UKCC. The procedure is called an application for judicial review. This is the procedure whereby a group of consultants unsuccessfully challenged Mr Kenneth Clarke's decision to spend money to implement

NHS changes before the relevant legislation had passed through Parliament, and whereby a former prostitute attacked an NHS infertility unit's decision to bar her from treatment.

5. High Court (Family Division)

The Family Division, as its name suggests, hears disputes relating to family relationships and breakdowns. For the nurse, its crucial role is in disputes over children, whether concerning allegations of abuse or genuine disagreements over treatment. In most child care disputes now, for example disputes relating to parental access after divorce or with whom the child should live, the Children Act 1989 defines the jurisdiction and powers of the court. But that Act preserves a wide discretionary power for the High Court (the inherent jurisdiction) and this power may be invoked in disputes over medical care such as whether the child of a Jehovah's Witness should be given blood transfusions regardless of parental objections.

6. Industrial tribunals

Industrial tribunals are not courts as such but specially created tribunals which consist of a qualified lawyer as chairperson and two lay members (representing employers' organisations and trade unions). They hear claims for unfair dismissal and for racial or sexual discrimination. Appeals on a point of law may be made to the High Court.

7. Coroner's Court

The coroner is a qualified lawyer or medical practitioner who enquires into sudden or suspicious deaths. The aim of the enquiry is to identify the deceased, the cause and place of death. So, for example, where a patient under your care commits suicide the coroner will investigate the death by calling witnesses and examining evidence.

8. The European Court of Justice

As a member of the European Community the UK is now subject to the law of that Community. The treaties upon which the European Economic Community was founded are incorporated into English law by the European Communities Act 1972. The European Court of Justice judges on Community law disputes. European Community legislation and case law are generally concerned with matters of trade and commerce and ensuring fair competition within member states.

The Community can enact legislation which has the same immediate effect as a British Act of Parliament. These forms of legislation are called *regulations*. Examples of Community regulations include detailed rules on food and other product standards. More usually the Community regulates by way of *Directives*. The Directive sets out a common European policy and requires member states to legislate to implement that policy. An example of such a Directive is the Product Liability Directive of 1985 implemented into English law by the Consumer Protection Act 1987. That Act provides that producers are 'strictly liable' for unsafe products. This means you do not have to prove that the production process was negligent. Other Directives relevant to nurses include those concerned with equal pay and mutual recognition of professional qualifications. EC law ought ultimately to enable you to practise as a nurse in any European Community State. Disputes arising out of EC legislation will ultimately be heard in the European Court of Justice. A judgment from that court binds all English judges.

9. The European Court of Human Rights

The European Court of Human Rights seeks to enforce the individual's human rights laid down in the European Convention on Human Rights. That Convention is a treaty agreed by many European nations, not just the members of the EC, and is quite separate from the European Community. The Convention is not immediately applicable in England but an unhappy litigant in England who has been all the way to the House of Lords, or as far as he or she can get, may appeal to the Court of Human Rights. However, judgments made in the Court of Human Rights are not directly enforceable in England. An adverse ruling against the law of England only shows disapproval of the current state of English law – in order for the judgment to have any effect the Government has to change the law, and the only sanction for not doing so is suspension from membership of the Council of Europe, the body enforcing the treaty. As the Convention of Human Rights deals with such matters as rights to life and to start a family, it can be very pertinent to ethical dilemmas in health care.

Law and morality

So far in this chapter on nurses and the law we have examined how law is made and looked at the courts which administer the law. But how should law be made? Nursing practice touches on the most sensitive and intimate issues of life and death. For example, laws on abortion require us to decide how we value the foetus. Is it a person like you, or is it simply a biological artefact? At the other end of life, is your life yours to end when you see fit or is it a gift from a Creator who decides the day it should end? Health professionals cannot escape the debate on the proper relationship between law and morality. Law and morality share a similar vocabulary. Both speak of rights and duties and the issues addressed are often one and the same. But the meanings assigned by the lawyer and the ethicist to similar words can be radically dissimilar. Nor does it follow that a moral obligation should necessarily be enforced by a legal duty. Most importantly in modern society there is often no consensus on morality, and your moral view may differ from mine. The law applies universally. Does it/ should it enforce your morality or mine?

A few examples will help to clarify this awkward relationship between law and morals. Beneficence (doing good) is, as we have seen, a key principle of ethical behaviour for the nurse. In both our professional and personal lives we might agree that we ought to try to do good to help others. Yet the law largely restrains itself to stopping bad conduct, to enforcing non-maleficence. You will be found liable in the tort of negligence if you carelessly inject a patient with an overdose of a drug, and if you are grossly negligent you might even go to prison for manslaughter. But if you witness a road accident and stand by while the victim dies for lack of simple measures well within your competence the law will not condemn you. You may have acted immorally, but the law will not compel you to be a Good Samaritan. Just because you are a nurse you are not legally obliged to be better than the rest of us. If you think the law should be more concerned with making people good, rather than just stopping us being bad, consider how far you would go. Should people be compelled to be blood donors? If your brother is dying of renal failure should the law order you to give him a kidney?

At least in the above example we all agree more or less on the question of morality. Where there is no such agreement the law/morality debate becomes even more tricky. In nursing the fundamental problem is often the sanctity of human life. Traditional Judaeo-Christian morality dictates that life from conception until natural death is sacrosanct. Abortion and voluntary or involuntary euthanasia are therefore prohibited to believers. Modern moral philosophers argue that human life as such has no value. Only persons capable of valuing their own existence have moral status. Killing the foetus is thus not immoral. Conventional sexual morality dictates a monogamous marriage relationship and condemns homosexuality, but those precepts are now rejected by many of us. How does the law then cope with issues like surrogacy or demands by homosexuals to assisted conception?

The Hart–Devlin debate

Does society have the right to pass judgment on matters of morality? Should there be a public morality or are morals a matter for private judgment? If society has the right to pass judgment does it also have the right to use law to enforce it? If so, should it use the law in all cases or only in some? And if only in some, on what principles should it distinguish? These questions were posed by the eminent judge Lord Devlin in examining the relationship between law and morality.

Devlin advocated the legal enforcement of morality. The morality that he suggests should be enforced is the 'shared morality' of the society in question. For him, this 'shared morality' comprises standards of conduct which are approved by the reasonable man. Devlin defines his average man rather more specifically, as being one whom law-makers recognise as immediately accepting the moral correctness of the laws laid down at any particular time. He cannot be a person who disagrees with the law because if he does so he, by definition, does not share the common morality. Devlin's reasonable man is therefore someone who agrees with the law as it is!

Devlin maintained that firstly, society has the right to pass judgment on morals because a society consists of individuals with a common or shared morality. Secondly, society does have the right to use the law to enforce morality in the same way as it uses law to safeguard anything else that is essential to its existence and that it values. 'Thus the suppression of vice is as much the law's business as the suppression of subversive activities.' His one proviso was that the law should only be used judiciously so that the privacy of individuals may be respected. He suggested that any behaviour which is tolerated by society should not be punished, although the level of tolerance will vary from generation to generation. For Devlin, the law is concerned with a minimum standard of behaviour and it is morally correct for the law to enforce this minimum standard of a particular shared morality.

Hart, an equally eminent professor of law, took a different view. He maintained that it is not permissible to enforce morality through law and that morality and law provide two distinct sets of rules to regulate behaviour. Instead of imposing a particular morality he argues for the freedom of individuals to do what they want provided they cause no harm to anyone else. He opposes legal intervention based solely on intolerance of particular activities and values individual freedom more than Devlin. Where people are distressed by the knowledge that others are behaving in an 'immoral' way, this, for Hart, does not constitute harm.

Despite differences the two views share some common ground. Rules, whether legal or moral, are necessary for the functioning of society. Legal rules are more coercive than moral rules in that breaches of the law can result in loss of liberty or loss of personal property. Both Hart and Devlin see the law as an instrument which should be used in some instances but not necessarily in others. They disagree on where and how you draw the relevant boundaries.

Individual and even 'shared' morality can differ so much that it is hard to say that law does or should enforce morality. Within your profession as a nurse you will often find that the legal rules applied are not as problematic as the ethical duties laid down. You may have no legal duty to be a Good Samaritan, but if you did ignore the needs of an accident victim you might be condemned by the UKCC and fellow professionals. Where nursing is concerned, the profession's moral view of a particular activity may well influence the law when it applies the standard of the reasonable or average nurse.

Conscientious objection

What if your personal moral code conflicts with 'shared morality' or some specific instruction which you are given as a professional? Where a nurse objects to performing a certain task because his individual morality causes him to, he may think that he has a right to conscientious objection. '. . . a true conscientious objector must think it would be morally preferable not to perform a required act even if no exemption were afforded for conscientious objectors and enforcement against him were certain' (Greenwalt).

Two specific rights of conscientious objection are granted under the Abortion Act 1967 (a right to refuse to participate in an abortion), and the Human Fertilisation and Embryology Act 1990 (a right to refuse to participate in any treatment covered by the Act). Where no specific right is given, the law and morality debate is extended. Do you have a right to disobey a law which you disagree with or feel to be morally wrong?

Conscientious objection is only one of many reasons for withdrawing from duties and obligations. Because there are so many different reasons it is impracticable for the law to list categories of exemptions which allow people to withdraw their services. A further problem for the law in dealing with conscientious objectors is that the usual methods of punishment are often inappropriate for the conscientious objector – imprisonment probably will not encourage the objector to reassess his beliefs! The very fact that the objector holds some firm belief may actually generate sympathy from others instead of condemnation.

In general the law does not provide a right of conscientious objection beyond the two exceptions listed. Since the law makes no provision for conscientious objection there would appear to be a conflict between the law and the particular conviction or morality in question. The obvious remedy for a conscientious objector is to avoid employment in a field or locality where they know they will be required to perform that specific treatment regularly. On a one-off occasion you should state your objection to managers, giving enough time for alternative arrangements to be made, but according to the UKCC advisory document *Exercising Accountability* a nurse must never refuse emergency treatment. And even the right to refuse to participate in abortion is limited by a duty to act where a mother's life is endangered.

Wherever there is a duty to act, an omission to do so may be actionable but as long as the patient receives the necessary care from somebody she will have no action against the objector for his omission. If, however, the objector were the only person available or if he refused in an emergency situation, the patient or her dependants might have some cause of action. More likely, the health authority would be sued for negligent performance of their duty to provide reasonable and adequate health care but the nurse may face disciplinary action if his employers decide that he is not complying with implied terms in his contract.

Such objections relate to the nurse's own conscience or beliefs. An objection, however, may arise where there is dispute between health professionals over the suitability of a particular course of action. For example, a nurse does not regard what is to be done as immoral, just poor practice. In this situation good practice should demand that the matter is discussed and any final decision should be made in the patient's interests. If after discussion the nurse still refuses to comply with, for example, the medical practitioner's prescription or decision, the nurse should make a record of his objections. In such a case his employers would make decisions about his objections and the law would probably only be implemented in relation to his contract of employment.

Conclusion

It is important to realise that fortunately although nurses are rarely sued or prosecuted personally, the law still plays an important role in your life as a nurse. The UKCC may have primary responsibility for regulating nurse conduct but the UKCC is subject to the law. Guidance from the UKCC on the nurse's obligations will be respected by the courts but ultimately the courts are the final arbiters of the legality of a nurse's behaviour.

4

Autonomy and consent

Act always in such a manner as to promote and safeguard the interests and well-being of patients and clients. (Clause one. *Code of Professional Conduct*)

The word autonomy is derived from Greek and literally means 'self-rule'. Autonomous beings have a type of freedom to control their lives which differs from non-autonomous beings. People are thought to be autonomous beings, as by reasoning they have the ability to make choices and exercise control over their lives. Non-autonomous beings such as animals may also be said to have freedom (providing they are not kept in a zoo), but an inability to reason means that they are not able to control their lives in the same way as autonomous beings. If we consider people to be autonomous beings, then this has implications for the sort of treatment they may expect from health professionals. So patients may expect to be fully informed of any diagnosis made and methods of treatment available, in order to exercise their right to consent to or refuse such treatment. Respect for patient autonomy is a crucial principle of nursing ethics. But just what does that principle entail and how does it work in practice?

Respect for autonomy

It may seem obvious that health professionals should fully inform a patient about his diagnosis, discuss the forms of treatment available and obtain his consent to the treatment proposed, because to act otherwise is to disregard the patient as an autonomous being. It is trite now to assert that patients have a right to give an 'informed consent'. To say that health professionals such as nurses should have respect for a person's autonomy, however, has wider implications than this. If we accept that an autonomous person, having been presented with the facts, makes a rational decision about the sort of treatment they want, then in order fully to respect that person's autonomy, nurses must accept whatever decision the patient makes. This can cause conflict for a nurse between her concern for a patient's well-being and respect for whatever decision the patient may come to, as, for example, when a person refuses life-saving treatment because of a religious belief, or when a person attempts to commit suicide. More complicated situations arise with individuals incapable of making a rational decision, such as babies, children and the mentally impaired. Who should make decisions about treatment on their behalf?

Perhaps respect for patient autonomy cannot be an absolute principle. What is important is to identify in what circumstances (if any) health professionals are justified in rejecting a decision made by a patient. The following case studies help to illustrate some of the problems in actually implementing respect for autonomy.

Sylvia's right to say no?

Sylvia Cavendish is sixty-eight and has suffered from rheumatoid arthritis for thirty years. Three years ago she developed peripheral vascular disease in her legs, which was treated by inserting an arterial graft. Following surgery Sylvia believed that the vascular disease had been cured and she was able to return to living on her own despite severe rheumatoid arthritis.

During the last eighteen months, however, Sylvia has become more disabled as a result of the arthritis, and her family became anxious about her living on her own. Sylvia and her family decided that Sylvia should sell her home and move to a private nursing home. Soon after moving into the home, Sylvia fell and sustained a fracture to her right humerus which was immobilised in a plaster cast. Sylvia had earlier accepted her change of lifestyle with resignation. She spent most of her day knitting and doing puzzles, but as she is right-handed the plaster cast made it impossible for her to continue such activities. The plaster also meant that Sylvia now had to rely heavily on the nursing staff for assistance to fulfil her basic needs. She found it difficult to accept a further loss of her independence.

Six weeks ago Sylvia began once again to show signs of peripheral vascular disease, and her GP requested a surgical opinion. The surgeon visited Sylvia and said that he suspected that the arterial graft had blocked. The only treatment possible was to amputate her right leg. The following day Ann Palmer, a registered nurse, visited Sylvia to discuss the proposed surgery with her. Sylvia said that she did not want to have her leg amputated and that she would refuse to give consent to surgery. Ann explained that the disease was life-threatening but Sylvia remained adamant about her decision. She told Ann that she knew that her fractured humerus was not healing, and that consequently she almost certainly would not regain the same use of her right arm as she had prior to her fall. Sylvia said that she had thought carefully about the surgery and had decided that she did not want to live if she could not maintain an acceptable degree of independence.

Ann was horrified that Sylvia should refuse what she saw as life-saving treatment. She felt that as a nurse she could not stand back and watch a patient die unnecessarily. Ann wondered if Sylvia was suffering from depression which had affected her judgment and so decided that she should try to persuade Sylvia to change her mind, or even find a way for the surgery to be carried out even if Sylvia continued to refuse to consent.

John's right to know?

John Wells, aged sixty-four, had recently undergone abdominal surgery when it was discovered that he had carcinoma of the stomach. It was not possible to remove the tumour, and there was evidence of metastasis in the liver. Mr Strong, the surgeon, carried out a procedure to bypass the stomach, which means that it will still be possible for John to tolerate some solid food.

Mr Strong is a consultant surgeon with many years' experience of treating patients with cancer. He believes that it is a mistake to tell patients that they are dying unless they are in the final stages of a terminal illness. Mr Strong thinks that John Wells will have approximately six months to live, which he will enjoy if he believes the operation has cured him. In Mr Strong's experience, a patient told that he has only six months to live gives up and wastes the last months of his life.

Sarah Gaskin is a staff nurse on the ward where Mr Strong's patients are cared for. Sarah has been allocated as John's primary nurse and, during the time he has spent in the ward, Sarah has got to know him and his family quite well, although, at first, he did not show any desire to discuss his diagnosis with her.

Two weeks after surgery, John is still feeling unwell although he has been reassured by Mr Strong that he is making good progress. John then tells Sarah that he thinks that he has cancer and that Mr Strong has not been telling him the truth. He asks Sarah directly if he does have cancer and if the operation has completely cured him. Sarah believes that Mr Strong is misguided in his views, but respects his position as an experienced consultant surgeon. However, she is dismayed by John's direct question and, as his primary nurse, Sarah feels that she should be able to give John information about his prognosis if he requests it. Sarah knows that if she tells John the truth he is likely to lose confidence in Mr Strong, and that she will also incur Mr Strong's wrath for deliberately going against his policy. What should Sarah do?

Paternalism

Both case studies beg the question of whether paternalism on the part of health professionals can be justified. Health professionals' genuine concern for the well-being of patients may in some cases cause them to demonstrate paternalism towards their patients. Paternalism means to believe that it is right to make a decision for someone without taking into consideration that person's wishes, or even to override their express wishes. As its name suggests, paternalism resembles the way parents may reach a decision about a child. Autonomy is overridden, but any action taken is thought to be in the child's best interests. In clinical practice, paternalistic decisions may be taken about a patient's medical treatment or nursing care without fully discussing the alternatives with the patient, or even by rejecting a decision that a patient may have reached and acting contrary to their wishes.

Health professionals may act in this way because of a belief that the patient has insufficient specialist knowledge to enable them to make an informed decision. Consequently they believe it is better to leave these sorts of decisions to well-informed health professionals. Another area of clinical practice where health professionals may fail to respect the patient as an autonomous being concerns telling the truth. In some circumstances, health professionals think it right to conceal the true diagnosis from a patient especially when the prognosis is poor. One justification advanced for acting in this way is that it may be difficult to ascertain whether patients do truly want to be told that there is no further treatment possible for their illness, and that death will not be long delayed. In cases of doubt, health professionals tend to err on the side of caution.

The dilemma in such cases is that respect for autonomy appears to conflict with the principle of beneficence and, to a lesser degree, the principle of non-maleficence, which have long and ancient traditions within medicine. Health professionals would agree that they have an obligation to do good, or at least to do no harm as far as patients are concerned. However, if doctors or nurses accept those principles as their primary obligations towards patients, respect for a patient's autonomy takes second place. Thus there is a danger in believing that beneficence should always override autonomy. It is well known that to be healthy a person should not smoke or drink excessive amounts of alcohol, should have a good diet, and take regular exercise. If health professionals believe that their overriding obligation is to act in their patients' interests, then should they ensure that patients follow these rules irrespective of whether they want to or not, and perhaps even use force if necessary to make the patients comply? After all, they are acting in the patient's best interests. Autonomous decisions are important for individuals in society and it is doubtful that even beneficent health professionals themselves would agree to such a strategy. It seems then, that a belief that one is acting in a person's best interests is alone an insufficient reason for overriding autonomy, and more cogent justification is necessary if autonomy is to be curtailed.

The limits of autonomy

Autonomy, the right to choose for yourself, deserves protection because of the potential for abuse once the principle is disregarded. Absolute respect for autonomy may not be practical. None of us always acts in every respect on full information and in the exercise of a true, unfettered choice. At any one time there will be several categories of people incapable of making any sort of decision for themselves. Perhaps what we should aim to achieve is respect for choices that are as autonomous as possible in the circumstances.

Harris in *The Value of Life* suggests that a person's decision may be considered as autonomous as possible if the following criteria are met:

1. That there are no apparent defects in control. For example, the person is not suffering from mental illness or drug addiction so that their choice is dictated by the illness or addiction rather than any reasoning process. Do anorexics suffer from a defect in control?
2. That there are no apparent defects in reasoning. The person is able to support their decision with adequate reasons for doing so, even though others may disagree.
3. That there are no apparent defects in the information available. For example, has the person been given inaccurate or inadequate information, or even been deliberately deceived?

If there are defects in a person's control, reasoning or the information available, that individual's ability to make an autonomous decision is undermined. By following these criteria, a nurse might only be justified in overriding a patient's choice because she could demonstrate that there was a defect in the autonomy. The decision was not a truly autonomous choice. If the nurse is unable to do this, what moral justification has she for her action?

Sylvia and John

Let us now go back to the two case studies. Sylvia decided that she did not want to have her leg amputated. Ann was amazed by that decision and felt that Sylvia had not made the right choice. What ethically can she do? Ann first needs to decide if Sylvia is capable of making such a decision by herself. Was Sylvia's decision autonomous enough?

Sylvia has not shown any signs of mental illness up to this point. She has managed to live adequately at home on her own despite being very disabled with arthritis. This does not suggest a person with mental illness. Sylvia decided herself that she could no longer go on living alone and made an autonomous decision to enter the nursing home in the first place. Taking all this into consideration, there do not appear to be any defects in control.

Ann might be justified in trying to limit Sylvia's autonomy if she could demonstrate that Sylvia was mistaken in her perception of the outcome of the amputation, that there is a defect in reasoning. The crucial issue is Sylvia's perceived loss of independence. Sylvia believes that an amputation would increase her dependency on others; she is obviously well informed about her illness and realises that having suffered for so long with arthritis, her fractured humerus is unlikely to heal satisfactorily which will also increase her dependency. It seems that Sylvia's reasoning is correct, as it is unlikely that the outcome of the surgery will be any different from her expectations.

Ann's final consideration should relate to the quality of information that Sylvia has been given. Suppose Sylvia has been misinformed, and that the surgeon only intends to remove the toes from her foot and not the whole leg. If this was so, Sylvia's choice was not truly autonomous and Ann should ensure that Sylvia is given the correct information about the amputation. Once that is done, if Sylvia considers that even that will affect her independence and still refuses to consent to the surgery, Ann has no alternative other than to consider her decision as autonomous.

The case of Sylvia illustrates the conflict between beneficence and autonomy. Ann wants to do what she perceives is right for her patient, to prolong her life. Sylvia wants to live as independently as possible. She does not value merely being alive with little independence. If Ann cannot show that Sylvia has not made an autonomous decision, she cannot justify overriding Sylvia's autonomy on grounds of beneficence alone.

In John's case, there are two issues to consider, firstly whether it is right to deceive patients about their prognosis and secondly, whether Sarah should comply with a decision about which she has misgivings.

Mr Strong clearly believes that the principle of non-maleficence is of primary importance, and as a consequence does not treat John as an autonomous being. Mr Strong considers that he should do the best for his patients, which in John's case would be to cure him of the cancer. If that is not possible, then he should at least do no harm. Mr Strong honestly believes that he is acting as an experienced clinician and according to the Hippocratic Oath. But as we have seen, acting in a person's best interests does not of itself justify overriding that person's autonomy. Even if it is true that some patients give up when told they have only a limited time to live, will it be true in every case? In some circumstances it may be essential that a person is told the truth, for they may have affairs (practical and emotional) which need to be dealt with before they die. The difficulty is deciding who does want to be informed of their prognosis and who would prefer not to be told.

Mr Strong is deliberately deceiving John. It is difficult to see this sort of deception as being morally different from telling lies. Mr Strong must therefore not simply justify not telling John the truth, but justify deliberately lying to him. Are health professionals bound by the same sort of moral codes as the rest of society? If telling lies is usually morally indefensible, can health professionals claim any special justification for deliberately lying to their patients? This is a particular dilemma for Sarah because she has been directly questioned by John regarding his condition. It would be plausible for her to assume that John really does want to be told his prognosis.

The fundamental difficulty for Sarah is whether she should lie to John even though she knows that it is morally indefensible, or contradict the consultant's usual policy of withholding information. The *Code of Professional Conduct* states that the nurse should: 'Act always in such a manner as to promote and safeguard the interests and well-being of patients and clients.' Sarah has to decide if telling John the truth in response to his direct questioning is acting in accordance with the *Code of Professional Conduct*, and if this is the case, then she must disregard Mr Strong's policy and risk his wrath.

In its document *Exercising Accountability*, the UKCC states that: 'Accountability can never be exercised by ignoring the rights and interests of the patient or client.' Sarah's position as an autonomous practitioner is threatened by Mr Strong. The UKCC seems to suggest that, in response to direct questioning, Sarah should tell John the truth. But this could cause conflict between professionals and that would not in the long term be in the patient's interests. Conflict between professionals is unfortunately quite a common occurrence in clinical practice and we discuss this more fully in Chapter Seven.

The problem of suicide

If you recognise patient autonomy as an important principle then it becomes very difficult to justify intervening when a person makes an autonomous decision to commit suicide. Might Sylvia by refusing life-saving treatment be seen as committing suicide? Her decision was as autonomous as possible, so the nurses caring for Sylvia can justify respecting her wishes and, we would argue, are ethically obliged to do so.

The situation is less clear when health professionals are faced with an attempted suicide in a hospital accident and emergency department. They may be unable to ascertain if the person's decision to die was made as autonomously as possible. Some individuals make as autonomous a decision as possible to commit suicide and truly intend to die. Others attempt suicide as a direct response to a crisis in their life and do not seriously intend to die. Theirs is a 'gesture' suicide. Others attempt to commit suicide, when they are unable to make a truly autonomous decision to do so in the first place, perhaps because of mental disorder. The difficulty is that patients who have attempted suicide are often unconscious and unable to tell you what their intentions were. When there is doubt about whether the person wishes to die or not, then health professionals are morally justified in intervening and saving that person's life.

One way of justifying that view is by using an example of John Stuart Mill. Suppose you saw someone starting to cross a bridge that you knew was unsafe, but there was no time to warn the person. Your only way of saving the person is to rush after him, seize him and bring him off the bridge. Although you are preventing the person carrying out his autonomous choice, that is to cross the bridge, you may be justified in doing so, because he may be unaware of the danger. This is similar to emergency treatment carried out to save the life of the person who has attempted suicide. If that person is unable to tell you what his intentions are, then in a similar way to the person crossing the bridge, health professionals may intervene and provide emergency treatment. However, this does mean that if the person's life is saved, and he is subsequently able to demonstrate that he has made as autonomous a decision as possible about ending his life, then the justification for intervention will no longer be possible should the patient refuse further treatment.

Consent

Consent to treatment is the means by which the patient exercises autonomy. Health professionals are obliged to disclose information to patients to enable them to make a decision as to whether or not to consent to any form of recommended treatment. In current practice the emphasis has shifted from health professionals being obliged simply to disclose information, to ensuring that the quality of information which a patient receives really enables him to make an autonomous decision. It is not enough simply to ask a patient if he will consent to a particular operation or use of a certain drug without explaining all the options that are available, and the consequences of each form of treatment. Health professionals usually have a greater knowledge about these matters than the patient and so the latter needs help to reach an autonomous choice. The health professional must explain the facts to the patient using language the patient is able to understand. Information only leads to autonomous choice if the patient understands that information. 'Informed consent' without understanding is useless.

For many treatments, particularly surgery, it is the responsibility of the doctor to explain the procedure to the patient and obtain the patient's consent. However, there are many clinical situations when you as a nurse must seek the consent of the patient before carrying out a procedure, particularly an invasive procedure, for example an intramuscular injection. The UKCC states that in this case, the nurse's obligation is that she 'explains the intended test or procedure to the patient without bias and in as much detail (including detail of possible reactions, complications, side effects and social or personal ramifications) as the patient requires'.

In its document *Exercising Accountability* the UKCC goes on to say that if the patient asks no questions then the nurse should assess and determine what information the patient requires. There will be some patients who want to be informed of every small detail of the recommended treatment including rare side effects or adverse outcomes. If the nurse is directly questioned about such matters, then it is morally indefensible to withhold information from the patient.

It is more difficult to assess what information the patient requires when no questions are asked. Suppose you are about to give a patient an injection of Pethidine which has been prescribed for severe pain. It would not be enough simply to inform the patient that you are going to give him an injection and expect him to agree. If the patient does not ask any specific questions, then it seems reasonable that you should explain why the drug has been prescribed, where you intend giving it and what effects the patient is likely to experience as a result. Pethidine is likely to cause drowsiness, dizziness, nausea and vomiting in any person to whom it is administered, and even if the patient does not question you about the side effects, you should inform him about them because this is information that the patient needs in order to make an informed decision. The patient can then decide himself if being free of pain is more important to him than the potential side effects. It may be argued that explanation of these facts is part of the prescribing doctor's role, rather than that of the nurse, but as you, the nurse, are actually administering the injection, you should ensure that the patient is fully aware of the treatment he is about to be given. If the patient refuses the injection, then you will need to inform the prescribing doctor and further discussion with the patient will have to follow.

Legal principles

How does the law approach the ethical dilemmas inherent in respect for autonomy? The right to autonomy is recognised and enforced by English law, although lawyers more usually talk about the right to self-determination. Legal disputes about autonomy focus on the validity of any consent given to treatment and the circumstances in which treatment may lawfully be given without consent. As you will see, the law relating to consent is far from perfect.

Battery and assault

Any intentional touching of a person without consent constitutes the tort of battery, whether or not any damage results from the contact. If valid consent is given, there is no battery. The legal protection afforded by the tort of battery turns largely on the substance and meaning of consent. A patient whose valid consent has not been obtained can sue in the civil courts for compensation. In some cases a criminal prosecution for assault may also ensue. The relevance of battery in health care is that many forms of treatment, with the exception of the administration of oral drugs, involve direct contact with the body of the patient. If the nurse acts without the patient's consent, a battery will have been committed. Even when consent to an operation has been obtained, a battery will also be committed if, by mistake, a different operation is performed. In *Allan* v. *New Mount Sinai Hospital* (1980) a woman who asked to be injected in her right arm but was then injected in her left arm won damages in battery. In *Schweizer* v. *Central Hospital* (1974) the surgeon performed a back operation when the patient had consented to an operation on his toe and was held liable for battery. A clerical error caused the mistake. Such mistakes involve carelessness and so the patient could also sue in negligence. But the two torts are not the same and the patient may well prefer to sue in battery.

In battery the patient need only show that he has undergone treatment which he did not consent to. It is irrelevant that no harm or injury was suffered or that the treatment may actually have benefited the patient. Mrs Devi in *Devi* v. *West Midlands AHA* (1980) agreed to a minor gynaecological operation. The surgeon, upon finding that she had a ruptured womb, sterilised her. Her action in battery succeeded because she had not consented to the operation performed.

When a patient sues in battery he must prove that he did not agree to the treatment, and so careful records of what is said and done must be kept. The nurse as defendant is liable in battery for all damage which actually ensues from her action, however idiosyncratic the patient's reaction may be. In negligence you are only liable for damage which is reasonably foreseeable. Finally, a person who is found liable in tort for battery may also have committed a criminal offence of assault and may be prosecuted and punished.

For these reasons the courts are reluctant to hold health care workers liable for battery. The word itself carries a stigma. The connotation is that the defendant is morally culpable.

The legal meaning of consent

A patient's consent, whether written, oral or implied from the circumstances, renders a proposed treatment lawful. In practice a written consent form is normally provided before surgery. However, consent may be implied without the use of writing or even words as, for instance, when a patient rolls up his sleeve and holds out his arm to be vaccinated (*O'Brien* v. *Cunard S.S. Co.* (Mass. 1891)). Mere consultation with a doctor or nurse, however, does not mean that consent to treatment may be inferred.

The written consent is usually given by way of a standard form recommended by the Department of Health, and substantially revised in 1991. The standard form may be altered or amended to suit particular circumstances. The form itself does not constitute consent but is evidence of the patient's consent to the proposed treatment. The form will usually provide authority for any additional surgery which is necessary in order to save the life of the patient. Such written consent is not compulsory and its relevance becomes insignificant if the patient proves that, despite having signed the form, he did not understand the implications of its terms.

How much must you tell the patient?

So patient autonomy is afforded legal protection through the principle that any interference with the patient's body is lawful only if the patient's valid consent has been obtained. The classical statement of that principle was provided by Justice Cardozo in *Schloendorff* v. *Society of New York Hospital* (1914): 'Every human being of adult years and sound mind has a right to determine what shall be done with his own body; and a surgeon who performs an operation without his patient's consent, commits an assault' (p. 126). That statement must, however, be qualified. The legal protection afforded to autonomy relies heavily on how consent is defined. In order for the consent to be valid, must the patient know everything about the procedure he is being asked to consent to? How much must he be told and how much must he understand?

If a patient has expressly refused the treatment offered, or consent is obtained by purposefully deceiving him, or even if you accidentally carry out the wrong procedure, there is clearly no consent at all. In any of the above examples, your contact with the patient constitutes a battery. There are, however, many situations in which the circumstances are far less clear-cut. Consider the case study involving Sylvia Cavendish and Ann Palmer. Ann had the task of discussing the proposed amputation with Sylvia. Presumably, part of her duty was to explain the surgery and try to obtain Sylvia's consent. It is important that Ann knows what she is obliged to tell Sylvia and what information she is entitled to withhold. If she deceives Sylvia in order to get her to consent, a battery will be committed if the amputation goes ahead. As long as Sylvia is deemed competent and understands what risks she runs, she has a legal right to refuse treatment, even if that refusal will result in her death (*Re T* (1992)).

However, exactly what Ann tells Sylvia and *how* she goes about it may affect the decision Sylvia makes. Change the facts for a moment and imagine that Sylvia did consent to the amputation on the basis of her discussion with Ann. Now let us examine two rather different scenarios. First, on recovering from surgery Sylvia discovers that contrary to the information given her by Ann her whole leg has been amputated and not simply the lower leg below the knee. Second, the operation performed is exactly as described by Ann but a blood clot develops in the upper limb necessitating further surgery to amputate the whole leg. Ann knew but never told Sylvia that there was a 3 per cent risk of such an occurrence. In both scenarios the result as far as Sylvia is concerned is the same. She has lost her whole leg and was never properly advised about the consequences of surgery. But as we shall see, the legal outcome of any action Sylvia may take against the surgeon and/or Ann is likely to be very different. In the first scenario, there is clearly a battery. Sylvia never gave any consent at all to the removal of her leg above the knee. In the second, Sylvia gave consent albeit a consent based on inadequate information; it was not an 'informed consent'.

Informed consent: a legal doctrine?

Does English law recognise and enforce a doctrine of informed consent? The answer, as we shall see, is hardly at all. Across the Atlantic the picture is different. In the USA in 1957 it was held in *Salgo* v. *Leland Stanford Jr University Board of Trustees* that lack of informed consent could destroy the legal effect of an apparent consent so rendering the treatment in question a battery. That judgment, however, paled into insignificance compared to the finding in *Canterbury* v. *Spence* in 1972 that courts should define what constitutes informed consent by reference to the information a reasonable patient would consider crucial to his decision as to whether or not to agree to treatment. Patients, it was said, must be advised of all *material* risks and side effects relating to the proposed treatment. Material risk was defined as follows: 'a risk is material when a reasonable person in what the physician knows or should know to be the patient's position, would be likely to attach significance to the risk . . . in determining whether or not to forgo the proposed therapy' (p. 780).

Put these two judgments together and you have a doctrine offering comprehensive protection for patient autonomy, a true doctrine of informed consent. However, even in the USA by no means all the individual state courts took the same stance on informed consent. Some jurisdictions rejected the patient standard in *Canterbury* v. *Spence*, preferring to find that what patients should be told should depend on what the majority of professionals judge they ought to know. Others accepted the patient standard, but found that a failure to meet that standard did not invalidate the patient's consent altogether but did make the professional susceptible to a claim in negligence, to allegations that she had not given the patient adequate advice. The Canadian Supreme Court reviewed the American cases in *Reibl* v. *Hughes* (1980). Surgeons had failed to explain to a patient undergoing brain surgery that the operation itself carried a 10 per cent risk of precipitating a stroke and a 4 per cent risk of death. They had accurately informed him of what they wished to do and why. The Canadian court accepted the patient standard. Patients should be advised of those risks or implications of treatment which sensible patients would want to know. But the court rejected arguments that failing to offer that information destroyed the legal effect of the patient's consent altogether rendering treatment unlawful and a battery. The patient who suffers harm through inadequate advice should sue in negligence, not battery.

Now, as we noted earlier, battery is often a more favourable remedy for the patient. He does not have to prove that he suffered any actual harm and he can recover compensation for all the consequences of the unauthorised treatment. But a finding in battery is harsh for the professional. Consider again the case of Sylvia and Ann in the scenario where the latter failed to explain the risk of a blood clot and subsequent surgery. You may think that Ann acted wrongly and failed to respect Sylvia's autonomy, but do you think that she (or the surgeon) should be prosecuted for assault (or, in her case, inciting assault)?

The English courts have followed the Canadian example as far as liability for battery is concerned. The crucial judgment defining what patients must be told to ensure a valid consent is *Chatterton* v. *Gerson* (1981). The facts of the case are instructive. Miss Chatterton had suffered constant pain at a post-operative site. Conventional methods of pain relief failed to abate that pain. Dr Gerson then persuaded her to agree to an intrathecal injection of phenol in her spine to numb the site of the pain permanently. He carried out the procedure twice but that did nothing to relieve Miss Chatterton's pain and resulted in some permanent loss of sensation and mobility in her right leg. That loss of sensation and mobility was an inherent risk of the procedure, however carefully it was performed. Miss Chatterton claimed that Dr Gerson had never warned her of that risk and that consequently her consent was invalid and he had committed a battery on her. Mr Justice Bristow rejected her claim in battery. He said: 'In my judgment once the patient is informed in broad terms of the nature of the procedure which is intended, and gives her consent, that consent is real, and the cause of action in which to base a claim for failure to go into risks and implications is negligence, not [battery]' (p. 1013). The decision set a standard which has been followed since. Where the patient complains about a lack of information she can only pursue that complaint in negligence.

Negligence and informed consent

Miss Chatterton, however, also sued in negligence. And that second claim was equally unsuccessful. The English judge hearing her claim rejected the patient standard for determining how much information a patient should be given when deciding whether to agree to proposed treatment. The standard which professionals, nurses or doctors, are expected to attain derived, the judge held, from the judgment of Mr Justice McNair in *Bolam* v. *Friern Hospital Management Committee* (1957), which we discuss more fully in Chapter Seven. In that case the judge had ruled:

> A doctor is not guilty of negligence if he has acted in accordance with a practice accepted as proper by a responsible body of medical men skilled in that art . . . a doctor is not negligent, if he is acting in accordance with such a practice, merely because there is a body of opinion that takes a contrary view. (pp. 587–8)

As Dr Gerson had given Miss Chatterton as much information as other responsible doctors would choose to offer, he was not negligent. Other doctors might operate more open disclosure policies, but differences in professional practice did not of themselves render Dr Gerson wrong. Note the Canadian stance that the patient should be told what patients want to know is clearly rejected in favour of the professional standard. As long as the professional, doctor or nurse, adheres to a responsible professional practice, the law sanctions that behaviour. Informed consent looks like a dead duck.

The implications of the judgment in *Chatterton* v. *Gerson* for legal protection of patient autonomy mean it is scarcely surprising that further litigation ensued to try to reverse its effect. The landmark case of *Sidaway* v. *Bethlem Royal Hospital* (1985) went to the highest court in the land, the House of Lords. The facts of the case are these.

Mrs Sidaway underwent an operation on her spinal column intended to relieve persistent pain in her neck and shoulders from which she had suffered for some time. Two risks were involved in the operation, firstly, a 2 per cent risk of damage to the nerve root which might, if it materialised, render the operation futile; secondly, a less than 1 per cent risk of damage to the spinal cord which could result in partial paralysis. Mr Falconer, the surgeon, probably warned Mrs Sidaway of the first risk but not the second. We shall never know what actually happened as by the date of the trial Mr Falconer had died and the trial judge had to infer what probably happened in his discussions with Mrs Sidaway. Unfortunately that second risk of damage to the spinal cord resulting in partial paralysis materialised, leaving Mrs Sidaway severely disabled despite the fact that Mr Falconer performed the operation with proper care and skill.

Mrs Sidaway could not claim against Mr Falconer for negligent performance of the operation, so she attempted to bring a claim on the basis that Mr Falconer failed to warn her of all the possible risks inherent in the operation and was thus in breach of his duty. Mrs Sidaway, like Miss Chatterton, was trying to establish that she had not been given sufficient information to enable her to give an informed consent to the operation. The issue the court had to address was 'whether she should have been more fully informed'.

Her action was dismissed by the trial judge. The Court of Appeal upheld his decision and affirmed the *Bolam* test as applicable to medical advice. The House of Lords in *Sidaway* had the power to change the law in relation to what and how much a doctor or nurse should disclose to a patient and thereby assert the patient's right to play a more active role in his or her own health care. They could have found the *Bolam* test inapplicable to advice on whether or not to agree to treatment. Instead the Lords, with only Lord Scarman dissenting, upheld the Court of Appeal's decision and pronounced that the test of liability in respect of a doctor's (and a nurse's) duty to warn of inherent risks was that the doctor or nurse is required to act in accordance with a practice accepted at the time as proper by a responsible body of professional opinion. The doctrine of informed consent was categorically rejected and a paternalistic model of health care was given support.

How much information you must disclose to your patient is determined almost entirely by acceptable professional practice, though remember that this may be subject to variation over time. *Sidaway* was, strictly speaking, concerned with what information you should volunteer: 'We are concerned here with volunteering unsought information about risks of the proposed treatment failing to achieve the result sought or making the patient's physical or mental condition worse rather than better' (Lord Diplock, p. 659).

Is the legal position different if the patient asks specific questions, for example, John Wells in the second case study? Can Mr Strong's opinion that it is right to withhold information from patients in their own interests be justified legally? *Sidaway* does not directly address that question. However, Lord Scarman, who unlike the other judges argued that normally patients should be told whatever a reasonable patient would want to know, does expressly allow for a defence of therapeutic privilege. A health professional, argues Lord Scarman, may lawfully withhold information which he believes may damage the patient's mental or emotional health. For the judges in the majority who uphold the professional standard as the norm, therapeutic privilege is less of a problem. As long as a reasonable body of professional opinion would withhold information in the patient's interest, no breach of duty to the patient has occurred. Providing Mr Strong can find sufficient support from his professional colleagues for his stance he is legally 'safe'. Sarah faces an ethical dilemma. The consultant has almost certainly acted lawfully, yet she may consider that she has an ethical obligation to tell the patient the whole truth.

There are some suggestions in the majority judgments in *Sidaway* that once patients positively seek information, the professional's duty to offer information may be expanded. Much emphasis was placed on evidence that Mrs Sidaway herself had not demonstrated any particular desire for detailed information about her proposed surgery. Could you argue that if a patient has positively demonstrated a wish for further information, there is a duty to provide that information? That was the argument advanced by the patient in *Blyth* v. *Bloomsbury AHA* (1985). Mrs Blyth, herself a nurse, asked several questions before agreeing to an injection of the long-term contraceptive drug, Depo-Provera. She suffered irregular bleeding and other side effects as a result of the drug and sued the health authority, arguing that the staff administering the drug gave her inadequate advice and information on which to base her decision to consent to the injection. The trial judge was sympathetic and ruled that when a patient expressly sought information he should be told all a reasonable patient in his circumstances would be likely to want to know. He adopted the patient standard. However, the Court of Appeal firmly overruled that judgment. 'Evidence directed to what would be the proper answer in the light of responsible medical opinion and practice fell to be placed in the balance.' Reasonable professional opinion, the court held, determines how patients' questions should be answered as much as how much information doctors and nurses should initially volunteer to patients.

Is there any difference in the legal duty to provide information to patients related to the nature of the treatment proposed? You might perhaps find it easier to regard a paternalist approach to a very sick patient facing complex and risky treatment for cancer as more acceptable than a similar approach in relation to a healthy woman making decisions relating to contraception. In *Gold* v. *Haringey AHA* (1988) Mrs Gold agreed to be sterilised immediately after the birth of her third child. She was not warned of the risk that, however carefully the operation is performed, occasionally nature repairs the damage and the sterilisation reverses itself. Nor, she claimed, was she advised that male vasectomy has a lower failure rate than female sterilisation. At the trial the evidence was that at the time Mrs Gold was sterilised, although some gynaecologists did expressly warn the patient of the risk of failure, others did not, preferring to stress the generally irreversible nature of the operation. So a body of professional opinion supported the defendant's restrictive disclosure policy. The judge found for Mrs Gold saying that there was no medical need for the operation, it was non-therapeutic treatment and so the patient standard should apply. But yet again the Court of Appeal intervened to assert that professional opinion and practice should *prima facie* determine what patients be told. If a procedure is carried out by a doctor or nurse, then providing he or she complies with a reasonable body of professional opinion in deciding what to tell the patient or how to answer his questions he or she has acted lawfully, in most circumstances.

You may by now have come to the conclusion that the law is more concerned with professional autonomy rather than patient autonomy. That conclusion should be treated with some caution, and two provisos must be stated straightaway. First, in *Sidaway* the House of Lords vehemently denied any suggestion that the judges were simply handing over control of what patients should be told to the doctors, granting doctors virtual immunity from challenge to their professional practices. Lord Bridge reminded health professionals that there might be cases where, even though no expert professional witness would condemn non-disclosure, a court might. He put it this way:

> I am of opinion that [a] judge might in certain circumstances come to the conclusion that disclosure of a particular risk was so obviously necessary to an informed choice on the part of the patient that no reasonably prudent medical man would fail to make it. The kind of case I have in mind would be an operation involving substantial risk of grave consequences, as for example the 10 per cent risk of a stroke from the operation as in *Reibl* v. *Hughes*. (p. 663)

So a completely, flagrantly unreasonable disclosure policy will be condemned even if professional opinion should sanction such a policy. However, such is the respect English judges hold for doctors that no such example of judicial condemnation of professional policy has yet surfaced clearly. Such are the hopes of aggrieved patients that they will no doubt continue to try to exploit this loophole in the professional disclosure standard asserted by *Sidaway*.

The second proviso to any universal application of the professional standard is this. While in *Hatcher* v. *Black*, forty years ago in 1954, Lord Denning appeared to sanction a 'therapeutic lie' in certain extreme circumstances, that view will be unlikely to prevail today. The law will require you as a nurse to tell the truth. It may not compel you to tell the whole truth, but a direct lie influencing the patient to accept treatment which he would otherwise reject will be likely to lead to legal liability, as well as ethical condemnation.

Two further points must be understood clearly to appreciate the law's approach (or withdrawal from) the doctrine of informed consent. First, in the unlikely event of an individual nurse being sued for negligence in relation to advice to a patient concerning treatment, remember that the crucial test of professional opinion is nursing opinion. The nurse is judged by what her peers consider proper and the difficulties faced by nurses in conflict with medical colleagues will be taken into account in formulating that opinion. Second, never forget professional opinion changes with the times. In *Gold* v. *Haringey AHA* professional opinion (in 1979) among gynaecologists sanctioned a very limited disclosure policy to patients considering sterilisation. Today the Royal College of Obstetricians and Gynaecologists, the Department of Health and virtually all other professional bodies require that doctors do tell their patients that sterilisation may very, very occasionally fail. A doctor sued over advice given in 1993 cannot say 'Oh well, I complied with policy in 1979 when I first became a consultant.'

The nurse and patients' rights

Nurses can often find themselves, as the case studies illustrate, in an awkward dilemma when the doctor has undertaken the task of explaining treatment to a patient and obtaining consent but the nurse feels that the explanation given is inadequate. Patients often feel more at ease with nurses and may be able to ask a nurse questions they did not put to the doctor. The importance of a nurse's role in protecting the patient's rights must not be underestimated. Clause one of the UKCC *Code of Professional Conduct* requires nurses to 'act always in such a way as to promote and safeguard the interests and well-being of patients and clients'. This could be interpreted in two ways. First, you could argue that in order to serve these interests, as a nurse, you should uphold patient autonomy and give substance to the patient's right to know. The second interpretation would allow the nurse to consider each case individually and decide that in some cases paternalism is acceptable and in others autonomy should be reinforced. But can a nurse substitute her judgment for that of the doctor?

The UKCC advisory document *Exercising Accountability* offers some guidance on nursing responsibilities in the domain of patient autonomy. The document imposes a duty of advocacy. Section D clause three says:

> If the nurse, midwife or health visitor does not feel that sufficient information has been given in terms readily understandable to the patient so as to enable him to make a truly informed decision, it is for her to state this opinion and seek to have the situation remedied.

Although the UKCC guidance is ethical guidance, their opinion is likely to be supported by the law because the nurse will be judged according to acceptable nursing practices. If the code is taken as setting the standard of creating a duty to protect patient autonomy and to inform the patient, then the law, one would hope, will uphold that standard. Such professional codes and advisory documents have received judicial recognition as representing acceptable professional opinion at any rate when they emanate from doctors. A recent example was provided in the House of Lords discussion on the withdrawal of artificial feeding and antibiotic care from a patient in a persistent vegetative state. The Law Lords agreed that the doctors involved had come to a decision that corresponded to responsible acceptable practice partly because their decision was in line with an advisory document issued by the BMA ethics committee.

Where the patient is incapable of consenting

What happens if a particular patient is incapable of giving any sort of consent to treatment? Must you stand aside and let the unconscious road accident victim bleed to death? Do you leave the elderly demented patient to suffer the agonies of his abscessed tooth? Of course not. The law provides principles and procedures relating to the authorisation or the treatment of mentally incapacitated patients. We deal with children in Chapter Nine and vulnerable persons in Chapter Ten. We look now at the unconscious patient.

Unconscious adults

Two separate predicaments must be considered. The first occurs when the patient consents to a particular operation but in the course of surgery, and due to unexpected complications in surgery, the surgeon decides that a further procedure needs to be carried out. Can that further procedure be carried out despite the lack of formal consent? The patient may have signed a consent form authorising any further necessary surgery. However, even if no such form was signed you may lawfully do whatever is truly necessary to save life. It is not sufficient justification that the treatment, though not necessary to save the patient's life, was in her long-term best interests. In *Devi* v. *West Midlands AHA* the patient had agreed to minor gynaecological surgery. The surgeon found a tear in the uterus and, deciding that a further pregnancy would endanger Mrs Devi's life, he went ahead and sterilised her there and then. He genuinely believed that he was doing what was best for her. None the less, immediate sterilisation was not necessary and he was found to have acted unlawfully.

The second predicament arises when a casualty patient is brought in unconscious. Nurses and doctors quite commonly involve relatives at this stage asking them to give proxy consent. Such consent is relevant only in demonstrating that the nurse's attitude was reasonable and that it might help to discover what the patient's wishes would have been. Strictly according to the law, once a person is eighteen years old no one else can consent to treatment on his or her behalf.

So what can you do? Imagine that you are on duty in casualty; a patient is brought in unconscious and it is evident that a blood transfusion is necessary. Ordinarily if you treated this person without consent your actions could be legally justified in one of two ways. The first way is to say that the patient's consent could be implied on the basis that if he were conscious he would probably consent to the saving of his life. The second way is to invoke the necessity principle again. In order to justify emergency treatment without consent the practitioner would have to prove that the intervention was reasonable in order to save the patient's life, or to prevent grave and permanent injury to his health. In this way giving the blood transfusion would be justified even though the patient was unable to consent. What if, however, someone who knew the patient well informed you that the patient was a Jehovah's Witness? You could not now contend that you believe that the patient would have consented had he been able to. Can you fall back on a defence of necessity? That depends on whether, in English law, the imperative to save life overrules any right to patient autonomy.

Consent, necessity and life-saving treatment

Let us look first at a Canadian case. In *Malette* v. *Shulman* (1988) a patient was rushed into hospital after a road accident. Nurses found a card, commonly carried by Jehovah's Witnesses, stating that in no circumstances was the patient prepared to accept blood. The card was signed, witnessed and of recent origin. The doctor on duty in the casualty department none the less went ahead and administered a blood transfusion. He was found liable in battery.

Compare that outcome to the recent English case of *Re T*. T had suffered serious injuries in a road accident when she was thirty-four weeks pregnant. A decision was made to deliver her baby by Caesarean section. Prior to surgery T, who was twenty years old, received a lengthy visit from her mother, a devout Jehovah's Witness. T was not a baptised Witness though she had attended Witness services. After her mother's visit she declared that in no circumstances was she to be given blood. She asked doctors if they had substitutes for blood and being told that there were such substitutes she signed a standard form refusing blood and exempting the hospital from liability for any consequences of not administering a transfusion. She underwent Caesarean surgery and a stillborn child was delivered. T lapsed into unconsciousness and her condition deteriorated badly. Prompted by her father and boyfriend, an application was made to the courts for a ruling on whether in the light of her refusal of blood, T could lawfully be given the transfusion necessary to save her life.

The Court of Appeal ultimately ruled T could be given blood. Lord Donaldson, the President of the Court of Appeal, confirmed that adult patients have 'an absolute right to choose whether to consent to medical treatment'. However, where life is at stake, if there is doubt about the reality of the patient's choice that doubt should be 'resolved in favour of the preservation of life'. In T's case the judges held firstly, that she was dangerously ill and heavily medicated when she made her choice – did she really know what she was doing? Secondly, her decision came only after a lengthy visit from her mother – was she subject to undue influence? Thirdly, she had insufficient information on the consequences of refusing blood. Doctors told her that there were substitutes for blood but did not explain their limitations. Indeed, the Court of Appeal severely criticised the hospital for the practice of getting patients to sign blood refusal forms designed primarily to protect the hospital, rather than inform the patient.

Re T does not conflict with *Malette* v. *Shulman*. In England as in Canada a competent patient can refuse even life-saving treatment, but the evidence that that truly is his choice must be unequivocal. Further confirmation that the patient's right of autonomy is absolute is provided by Lord Goff in the judgment that authorised doctors to stop treating Tony Bland (*Airedale NHS Trust* v. *Bland* (1993) (see further Chapter Twelve). He said:

> It is established that the principle of self-determination requires that respect must be given to the wishes of the patient so that if an adult patient of sound mind refuses, however unreasonably, to consent to treatment or care by which his life would or might be prolonged, the doctors responsible for his care must give effect to his wishes, even though they do not consider it to be in his best interests to do so . . . to this extent the principle of sanctity of human life must yield to the principle of self-determination. (p. 866)

Lord Goff's affirmation of the inviolable right to autonomy of an adult of sound mind clearly begs the question of how the law defines competence. What degree of learning disability, mental illness or confusion renders a patient incompetent? That matter will be discussed in Chapter Ten. In this chapter we must conclude with an examination of one scenario in which it has been judicially argued that even a competent patient's autonomy may be infringed. In Re T Lord Donaldson added one qualification to his assertion that an individual's right to choose for himself whether to agree to medical treatment was paramount: 'a case in which the choice may lead to the death of a viable foetus'.

Such a case came before the Family Division of the High Court in Re S (1992). S was six days overdue beyond her expected date of delivery and had been in labour for two days. The baby was in transverse lie and there was a serious risk that S's uterus would rupture if labour continued. The doctors described her condition as 'desperately serious'. S was a born-again Christian and, with the support of her husband, she refused on religious grounds to submit to a Caesarean section. The probable consequence of that refusal was that both she and the baby would die. The President of the Family Division granted the health authority a declaration that it would not be unlawful to carry out a Caesarean section. The baby in fact died *in utero* but the mother recovered. S's competence was not discussed. The judge did not base his order on a finding that S was so ill after her terrible labour that she could not make a rational judgment. The order necessarily depends on an assumption that once a foetus is viable its interests must be weighed in the balance and can in an appropriate case outweigh the mother's right to autonomy. Do you agree? In the USA court-ordered Caesareans are not uncommon. The majority relate to women from ethnic minorities, and several women for whom the court ordered an 'essential' Caesarean actually gave birth to healthy babies vaginally. Four years prior to *Re S* in *Re F (in utero)* (1988) the Court of Appeal had unequivocally refused to intervene to compel a mother to accept treatment doctors judged necessary in the interests of the foetus. The legal status of the foetus is discussed further in Chapter Eight.

Conclusion

Autonomy, or self-determination, on the part of competent patients is recognised in both ethics and law. Note that, for the nurse, her ethical obligation to respect and advance the autonomy of each individual patient may, in many instances, be a higher and more onerous duty than that imposed on her by law. The law demands, on pain of liability for battery, that she obtain the initial go-ahead for anything she does to a patient. Thereafter, in counselling and advising that patient she must conform to standard practice. Her ethical obligation involves a greater sensitivity to the needs of each patient. Ethicists and lawyers both now recognise in principle a right to refuse even life-saving treatment. Both groups struggle with the implications of that principle. Think about how you would apply the arguments in *Re T* if an unconscious patient is brought into casualty after a suicide attempt. Would there be sufficient doubt about his true intentions to justify treating him? What if there is a note pinned to his jersey stating, 'Do not save my life in any circumstances'?

5

Confidentiality and whistleblowing

Protect all confidential information concerning patients and clients obtained in
the course of professional practice and make disclosures only with consent,
where required by the order of a court or where you can justify disclosure in
the wider public interest. (Clause ten, *Code of Professional Conduct*)

The principle of confidentiality has a long tradition amongst health care professionals, and for doctors has its origin in the Hippocratic Oath. In support
'The law has long recognised that an obligation of confidence can arise out
of particular relationships. Examples are the relationships of doctor and
patient . . .' A.G. v. *Guardian Newspapers (No. 2)* (Lord Keith, p. 639,
1988). For nurses, respecting confidences is often seen as having two practical applications; firstly, respecting the confidences of the patient and,
secondly, respecting the confidences of colleagues.

Confidentiality and patients

During any sort of contact with health care professionals, patients may
disclose information about themselves which they consider to be secret.
This information is given on the understanding that the person to whom
the information is given will not divulge it without the consent of the
patient. The patient may directly disclose information to a nurse, or the
nurse may be aware of confidential information regarding a patient because of access to records. In either situation a nurse has a special duty to
consider such information as secret irrespective of how such information
was obtained.

Health professionals have a special duty to respect the confidences of the
patient as part of their professional responsibilities. This type of responsibility has been described by H. L. A. Hart as 'role responsibility'. Professor Hart suggests that if a person occupies a distinctive place or office
within society and as a result has duties attached to this position, then that
person is responsible for fulfilling whatever duties are recognised as part

of that role within society. This role responsibility is of course not restricted to professional roles and may include such examples as the responsibilities a parent has as regards rearing a child, or a secretary of an organisation has in keeping the minutes of meetings.

As nurses do not make specific promises or take an oath to respect confidences, you may wonder what the reasons are for recognising a special professional duty for doing so. One explanation for this uses a consequentialist approach. If a patient believes that health professionals will keep secret any information that is given to them, then the patient is more likely to give all relevant information freely. As the aim in giving such information in the first place is to initiate effective treatment, it is in the patient's interests to make sure that the person treating them has all the relevant facts. Therefore, by trusting health professionals with confidential information, the patient is more likely to be treated more effectively which in turn raises the standard of health and welfare of society in general.

Another explanation is that patients give health professionals information about themselves only on the understanding that they will keep it secret, therefore establishing a form of 'contract' between the patient and health professional. The fact that many people assume that their confidentiality will be respected as a matter of course, and that health professionals do have an obligation to keep secrets, supports this explanation. Others may consider that they have a right to privacy and that they alone have personal control over information about themselves and, therefore, whom they choose to allow access to it.

Nurses may accept that they have a duty to respect patients' confidences, but can it always be regarded as an absolute principle? Consider the following case studies.

The epileptic fire officer

George Dawson is a fire officer and one of his responsibilities is to drive a fire engine. His wife does not have a job because they have four small children, three of whom are under school age. George has recently been diagnosed as having epilepsy. He has been prescribed anticonvulsant drugs, and two months after his discharge from hospital, he visits Dr Thomas, his GP, for a repeat prescription of his medication.

While at the surgery, George meets Pamela, the practice nurse, and during her conversation with George she is alarmed to discover that George has not told the fire service that he has epilepsy and is still driving the fire engine. Pamela attempts to persuade George to inform his employers, but George thinks that there is a possibility that he will lose his job. If he does so, this will seriously compromise the family's finances. George begs Pamela not to disclose his diagnosis so that he can continue to work for the fire service. Pamela knows the family well, but feels that she has a responsibility to inform the DVLC (Driver and Vehicle Licensing Centre) that George has epilepsy and is therefore unfit to drive a vehicle.

The HIV positive mother

Carol Grant makes her first visit to her local hospital antenatal clinic when she is fourteen weeks pregnant. Staff Midwife Johnston, while recording Carol's medical history, discovers that there is a possibility that Carol may be infected with HIV and reports this to Ms Grey, the obstetrician under whose care Carol is booked. Ms Grey discusses this possibility with Carol, and in view of the potential risks to the foetus, Carol agrees to a blood test to detect HIV.

Unfortunately this test proves to be positive, so Carol is informed of the result and counselling is given. Carol decides to continue with the pregnancy, but states that in no circumstances should her partner be informed of the fact that she is HIV positive. Midwives working in the clinic are unsure about complying with Carol's wishes and a case conference is called.

Staff Midwife Johnston suggests that the midwife's primary responsibility is to the client and her foetus and this includes respecting her confidentiality. She also states that it is common practice to record information in a client's notes that her partner is unaware of the fact that previous pregnancies have been aborted, or a child from an earlier relationship has been adopted. Sister Jones agrees with this, but feels that because Carol's partner is at risk of developing a potentially fatal illness, then he has a right to be informed even without Carol's consent.

Ms Grey considers that Carol's pregnancy will have to be very carefully monitored which may alert her partner to the fact that there are complications. Ms Grey wonders what she should say if she is directly questioned by Carol's partner about the pregnancy. She would be willing to withhold the information at Carol's request, but fears that if questioned about the pregnancy, in order to protect Carol's confidentiality she might be forced to lie to her partner.

Limits of confidentiality

If confidentiality were to be considered as an absolute principle, it would be necessary for the confidences of the patient to be kept, irrespective of the consequences of doing so. In some cases are there other, perhaps more important, factors to be taken into consideration? The following true case history from the USA shows how respecting the patient's confidence at all costs can have dire consequences (*Tarasoff* v. *Regents of the University of California (1976)*).

In August 1969 a student, Prosenjit Poddar, consulted Dr Lawrence Moore, a psychologist at the University of California. He told Dr Moore of his intention to kill his former girl friend, Tatiana Tarasoff. The police were informed of this and Mr Poddar was briefly detained, but he was later released when he convinced the police that he was of no threat to Tatiana Tarasoff.

Neither Ms Tarasoff nor any member of her family was informed of the potential danger she was in from Mr Poddar. Mr Poddar persuaded Ms Tarasoff's brother to share an apartment with him close to where Ms Tarasoff lived and, on 27 October 1969, Mr Poddar went to where Ms Tarasoff lived and killed her. Ms Tarasoff's parents brought a legal action against Dr Moore's employers, the University of California, for negligence in failing to warn Tatiana of the danger their patient posed to her.

Dr Moore obviously felt obliged to respect the confidences of Mr Poddar, and not disclose his intentions to Ms Tarasoff, even though her life was in danger. The difficulty in this case lies in deciding whether it was more important for Dr Moore to keep the information about Mr Poddar's intentions secret and therefore respect his confidences, or to be concerned about the safety of another individual. The case is complicated by the fact that Dr Moore could not assess exactly how serious Mr Poddar's threats were and so whether Ms Tarasoff really was in danger. Despite this difficulty, it may be assumed that Dr Moore did think that Ms Tarasoff was in danger as he took Mr Poddar's threats seriously enough to inform the police and have him detained. Therefore it would appear that Dr Moore faced a stark choice between either informing Ms Tarasoff of the threat to her life, or respecting the confidences of his patient, Mr Poddar.

As Dr Moore decided on the second alternative, it seems that he considered respect for confidentiality to be an absolute principle. You might think that in these circumstances, the prevention of Ms Tarasoff's murder was of overriding importance, even if in doing so Dr Moore disregarded his special duty to keep the confidences of his patients. And of course, even in this case the principle of confidentiality was not considered by Dr Moore to be absolutely inviolable because he did go to the police. That action weakened his case. Does it make sense to believe that he should respect Mr Poddar's confidences at all costs and at the same time be willing to inform the police of his threats?

Even though confidentiality cannot be thought of as absolute, it is still an important ethical principle and breaches of confidentiality must never be approached lightly. In their advisory document *Confidentiality*, the UKCC elaborates clause ten of the *Code of Professional Conduct*. Although the *Code* suggests that practitioners should disclose information if required by law, or if it is necessary to the public interest, the UKCC clearly considers that any breaches of confidentiality must be regarded as exceptional.

George and Carol

So in our two case studies, are the circumstances so exceptional as to justify breaching either George's or Carol's confidences? In the case of George, the fire officer, Pamela knows that by telling his employers or the DVLC about George's epilepsy she puts him at risk of losing his job and financial ruin. The obligation to respect George's confidence must be respected unless there are overwhelming reasons for breaking the confidence. By continuing to drive the fire engine, George is risking the lives of his colleagues, other drivers and pedestrians. Would Pamela be justified in seeing these interests as overriding, and informing the DVLC? After all, George may be unduly pessimistic about his work situation. It is possible that the fire service may still offer him other, more suitable, employment. Because of the magnitude of the risks involved, you might argue that Pamela is not only justified in breaching George's confidence, but has a moral obligation to do so. Such an obligation to disclose is not as readily recognised or discussed as the obligation to respect confidentiality. If a patient puts others at risk of serious harm, should an obligation to act to avert the potential danger be overriding?

In Carol's case, she is discovered to be HIV positive yet requests that her partner not be informed of this fact. A conflict of interests obviously emerges between protecting Carol's confidences and informing her partner of the health risk to him. As we saw, three opinions were given on how to respond to that conflict. Staff Midwife Johnston argues that she has a duty to protect the confidences of the client. It is true that it is common practice to record information that a client's partner may not be aware of, but the examples she uses are quite different to the circumstances of this case. The partner of the client who has had an abortion or a child adopted is not himself at any risk if this information is withheld from him. He is certainly not at risk of developing a potentially fatal disease as is Carol's partner. Her examples do not support her argument.

What advice would the nursing professional body offer? The *Code of Professional Conduct* states that disclosure of information without the consent of the patient is permissible if it is considered necessary in the public interest, defining public interest as 'the interests of an individual, or groups of individuals or society as a whole and would (for example) encompass matters such as serious crime, child abuse and drug trafficking'.

Sister Jones might argue that to inform someone that he is at risk of developing a potentially fatal illness should be considered as being in the interests of an individual as stated in the *Code*. It is left to the practitioner to decide what circumstances equate to serious crime, child abuse or drug trafficking. Sister Jones must reflect on whether the risk to Carol's partner really is sufficient to justify informing him of her HIV status. Sister Jones obviously felt that Carol's partner has a right to be informed, suggesting that she considered not merely that it was permissible to breach confidentiality in this case, but that she had a duty to do so, akin perhaps to Pamela's duty to prevent George continuing to drive.

Ms Grey, the obstetrician, seems to seek a compromise between the conflict of interests inherent in the case. Her response suggests that she sees a difference between deliberately withholding information from Carol's partner and lying to him should he question her directly. Does the compromise work? The key issue here is one of intention. As Ms Grey has full knowledge of the facts of the case, it could be said that even without saying anything false to Carol's partner she is still deliberately deceiving him. Is this sort of deliberate deception morally different from telling deliberate lies?

Ms Grey must decide if she considers it more important to respect Carol's confidences rather than to warn her partner of the risk to his health. If she decides that it is more important to protect her client's confidentiality, should she be prepared to do so in whatever circumstances arise, even if she is directly questioned? Ms Grey recognises a duty to respect confidences, and does not recognise a duty to inform as Sister Jones does. Logically it follows that, if Ms Grey considers that respecting her client's confidences is of overriding importance, she is faced with no alternative other than to lie to Carol's partner should he question her about the management of Carol's pregnancy. Consider what you would do if George or Carol were your patients. Try to answer the following questions for yourself. Do you agree that Pamela has a moral obligation to protect the public at large by informing the DVLC of George's medical condition? Which viewpoint in relation to Carol is closest to your own views on this case? How can your own views be defended with reference to clause ten of the *Code of Professional Conduct*? Is there a moral difference between deception and telling lies? Do you recognise both a duty to respect confidences and a duty to inform? If so, try to think of cases when one duty would be of greater importance than the other?

Legal principles and confidentiality

Ethical debate on confidentiality throws up difficult questions but few conclusive answers. How far does the law define the nurse's duty of confidentiality to his patients? The law does recognise and enforce a professional obligation of confidentiality. If you breach a patient's confidence, he may go to court and demand compensation from you and/or ask the court to forbid you to breach that confidence further. A court order, an injunction, is regularly used to restrain breaches of confidence in many spheres of activity. None the less in the context of health care patients complaining of breaches of confidence will often choose to complain to the health professional's regulatory body (e.g. the UKCC) rather than go to court. We shall see why this is a little later.

Lawyers argue endlessly about the precise nature of the legal obligation of confidentiality. What is clear is that such an obligation arises between the nurse and his patient whether the patient is treated within or outside the NHS. Breach of confidence is not a criminal offence in England, although it is in parts of Europe. The professional who betrays a confidence commits a civil wrong and will be ordered to compensate the patient for any ensuing damage as well as being prevented from committing further breaches of confidence. So, for example, if a nurse were to gossip to the local churchwarden about a sexually transmitted disease in respect of which he had treated the vicar, could the vicar sue the nurse if he lost his job?

An obligation to maintain confidentiality arises in law whenever the following apply:

1. A person entrusts to another information of a confidential nature.
2. The circumstances are such that it is obvious that the recipient is intended to keep that information secret.
3. It is in the public interest to safeguard the secrecy of that information.
4. Unauthorised breach of confidence will be damaging to the person confiding that information.

Once an obligation of confidence has arisen it applies as much to third parties to whom the confidence is imparted as to the orginal confidant. So if after clinic Dr X says to you 'Guess what – you'll never believe this, the vicar's got syphilis!', you are bound to keep that confidence even though it was not originally entrusted to you and even though Dr X acted improperly in telling you. The earliest known case concerning medical matters is from 1820, *Wyatt* v. *Wilson*, where action was taken against George III's physician to stop him from publishing his diary which contained information about the king's health and mental stability. A more recent example is *X* v. *Y* when in 1988 a judge prohibited a tabloid newspaper from identifying two HIV positive general practitioners.

Unfortunately the protection provided by the law for medical confidences may not always be terribly useful. The law is effective in aiding a patient who anticipates a breach of confidence, like the doctors who were alerted to the fact that the newspaper planned to reveal their HIV status in 1988. In such circumstances, if the patient goes to court and proves his case, he will be awarded an injunction to prevent the information from being disclosed and any relevant documents will be returned. However, the law is less useful once a breach of confidence has already occurred. The information will already be public so an injunction at this stage can only be used to stop any further disclosure. Redress is what the patient will be seeking.

Damages, to compensate the victim for monetary loss resulting from a breach of confidence, are a valuable remedy in cases which *usually* involve a breach of confidence in a trade or commercial context (e.g. an employee 'leaks' trade secrets to a competitor), where the loss suffered is foreseeable and measurable. When a medical confidence is breached, the injury or damage which the patient suffers is often likely to be embarrassment, annoyance or other mental distress. Such injury is hard to quantify and translate into a monetary award. The courts are hesitant about awarding compensation for such mental or emotional distress. The patient may go through the trauma and expense of a court case and get nothing for his pains.

Unsurprisingly, then, aggrieved patients remain more likely to make a complaint to the UKCC than start legal action against a nurse or doctor. The UKCC will focus on the propriety of the nurse's conduct as opposed to the patient's loss, and can impose the ultimate sanction by declaring a nurse unfit to practise. The cost of taking such a complaint to the UKCC is negligible when compared with the cost of a court action. However, just because the UKCC rather than the courtroom is the more likely forum to adjudicate on breaches of confidence, that does not mean the law is irrelevant. The UKCC itself is ultimately accountable to the courts and must take full account of how the law defines obligations of confidence and when the law will excuse or even compel a breach of confidence.

We have seen that the ethical obligation of confidentiality may on occasion be overridden by an ethical imperative to protect the interest of others. The law too recognises that obligations of confidentiality cannot be absolute but may have to be weighed against other interests. Consequently the law requires that nurses breach confidence in certain sets of circumstances, and leaves them free to do so in others. Let us look first at those situations where the law may demand that you breach your patient's confidence.

There are three principal sets of circumstances in which this may happen as follows:

1. Under general legislation.
2. Under health care legislation.
3. By an order of court.

In any of these cases where the law compels you to hand over information about patients, clause ten of the UKCC Code makes it clear that compliance with the law is not a breach of the nurse's professional ethical obligation.

1. General legislation
An Act of Parliament may demand that any citizen answer certain questions put by police officers or representatives of some other public authority,

e.g. in relation to road traffic accidents. The case which best illustrates this point is *Hunter* v. *Mann* (1974). Dr Hunter had information, acquired in his professional role, which might have led to the identification of a driver of a stolen car who was alleged to be guilty of dangerous driving. Under the Road Traffic Act a police officer may require any person to answer questions relating to such information. When questioned, Dr Hunter refused to divulge the identity of the person because he felt to do so would be a breach of his professional duty of confidence. The court held that a doctor acting within his professional capacity and carrying out his professional duty came within the words 'any other person' in the Act and therefore a statutory duty was imposed on him. He was convicted for failing to fulfil his statutory duty to, in effect, breach his duty of confidentiality. He enjoyed no special privilege just because he was a doctor. But the judges warned that in such a case a doctor or nurse should 'only disclose information which may lead to the identification and not other confidential matters'.

Does this mean that whenever a nurse has information that a criminal offence has been or may be committed she must inform the police? Suppose that George, the epileptic fire officer, told Pamela that he had killed someone while driving because of his epilepsy but until now no one knew. Is she obliged by law to contact the police? If she did not, would she be committing a crime? The simple answer is 'no'. There is no general obligation to volunteer information to the police (Criminal Law Act 1967 s.5(5)) except where a particular statute expressly creates such a duty. It is a criminal offence to lie to the police, or to accept money or a bribe, or to conceal evidence (s.5(1)). It is not a crime to stay silent save in the exceptional case provided for by anti-terrorism legislation. The Prevention of Terrorism Act, as amended in 1989, creates a criminal offence which is committed if any person fails to provide information which might lead to the prevention of terrorism and/or the apprehension of a terrorist. You need not contact the police if your patient tells you he broke his leg escaping from an attempted burglary. You must do so in the unlikely scenario when a patient confesses that his burns result from a bomb attack on the House of Commons.

2. Health care legislation

There are a number of statutes concerned with health care which require health professionals to disclose health care information about their patients, e.g. notification of certain infectious diseases. The supply of this information is supposedly for the general good of society, and some examples follow. The Public Health (Control of Diseases) Act 1984 requires that notification be made to the relevant local authority if a medical practitioner attends a patient with cholera, plague, relapsing fever, smallpox or typhus. AIDS is not yet a notifiable disease, but the Act empowers a local authority to direct that other infectious diseases be made notifiable. The Reporting of Injuries, Disease and Dangerous Occurrences Regulations 1985 have a similar purpose. Other obligations concern the collection of data, for instance, the Abortion Regulations 1968 SI 1968/390, and others provide information about those individuals who need state help such as the Misuse of Drugs (Notification of and Supply to Addicts) Regulations 1973 SI 1973/799.

3. By an order of court

In proceedings in court you may be ordered to give evidence including specific information about a patient to the court. Apart from specific statutory obligations of the sort just noted, you as a nurse should not normally disclose confidential information without the patient's consent unless ordered to do so by a court of law. If you are subpoenaed, i.e. your attendance in court is demanded, this order must be obeyed. Anything less, such as a request for information by a solicitor, need not be obeyed. Once in court you must answer questions posed. There is no privilege which entitles health care professionals (and other professional groups, including clergy, bankers and doctors) to refuse to give evidence on the basis of their professional relationship with their clients. The only relationship which enjoys such a privilege is that between a lawyer and her client! The only protection for confidences within the courtroom lies in the fact that the judge has a discretion to limit the amount of information which you will be ordered to disclose and is likely to be sensitive to the need to protect confidentiality as far as the needs of justice permit. If the judge decides that the questions must be answered, a refusal by you to comply with the order places you in contempt of court.

Voluntary disclosure of a patient's confidence

When the law compels you to disclose information and breach confidence with a patient, you may be unhappy to have to do so but at least your own legal responsibility is clear. You have to comply and neither the courts nor the UKCC can condemn you for your action. Far more difficult is the situation where no express legal duty compels you to breach confidence, but you judge that the interests of others outweighs your duty to the patient. You choose to disclose information 'in the public interest'. How does the law define that public interest? Clause ten of the UKCC *Code of Professional Conduct* gives as an example 'matters such as serious crime'. Could you argue that while not compelled to report evidence of any crime to the police you should, as a citizen, be free to do so? There is no clear ruling on the matter. Judicial opinion was split in the case of a doctor who had attended a woman (after she had had a criminal abortion) and then reported her to the police. One judge thought that such a breach of

confidence was inexcusable but another maintained that the most important duty was to 'assist in the investigation of serious crime'. In this century
the second opinion has tended to be followed. So, if Pamela informed the
police that George had killed a person and following that he was later
apprehended, it is unlikely that he would succeed against her in an action
for breach of confidence.

The nurse must do all that she can to obtain the patient's consent to
disclose the relevant information. Failing that, she must weigh her duty to
her patient against the risk of harm to other individuals. The UKCC, like
its medical counterpart the GMC, is clear that only matters of serious
crime justify breach of a patient's confidence. Reporting a patient's confes-
sion of shoplifting to the police will probably be unethical. The legal status
of such a disclosure remains unclear.

With luck, few of you will have to decide whether to contact the police
to report a patient's crime. More common, alas, will be situations like
those posed in the earlier case studies where your patient poses a risk to
the health and safety of others. When will the law excuse a breach of
confidence in such circumstances? First, if the patient later takes you to
court, the court decides whether breach of confidence is justifiable. In a
sense you disclose at your own risk. In addition to an action for breach
of confidence you may also be sued for defamation (libel or slander) if you
are mistaken about some of the information, and accidentally defame your
patient, by for example a false allegation that he is HIV positive.

The public interest defence and its effect on the duty of confidentiality

The key question for the nurse remains what sort of risks to others justify
invocation of the 'public interest defence' to an action for breach of confidence. The first point to remember is that the law recognises a strong
public interest in confidentiality. In several spheres of life, of which health
care is one, confidentiality is essential if people are to do 'business' together. So factors justifying a breach of confidence must be significant.
Lord Goff put it this way in A.G. v. Guardian Newspapers (No. 2) (1988):

> although the basis of the law's protection of confidence is that there is a public
> interest that confidences should be preserved and protected by the law, nev-
> ertheless that public interest may be outweighed by some other countervailing
> public interest which favours disclosure . . . It is this limiting principle which
> may require a court to carry out a balancing operation, weighing the public
> interest in maintaining confidence against a countervailing public interest
> favouring disclosure. (Lord Goff, p. 659)

To illustrate the actual working of this balancing operation let us look in
detail at two recent judgments concerning medical confidences.

In *X* v. *Y* (1988) an employee of the plaintiff health authorities gave information contained in hospital records to a tabloid newspaper. The information identified two doctors who had contracted HIV and still continued working in general practice. The newspaper published an initial article alleging that there were doctors who, in spite of contracting HIV, were continuing to practise and endangering patients. Their intention was to publish a further article identifying the two doctors.

The health authority sought an injunction prohibiting the newspaper from publishing the identities of the doctors. The court had to decide whether such a disclosure was justified in the public interest, as the newspaper maintained. In order to begin answering that question the court first had to identify all the interests at stake. This is how Mr Justice Rose approached the issue:

> on the one hand, there are the public interests in having a free press and informed public debate; on the other, it is in the public interest that actual or potential AIDS sufferers should be able to resort to hospitals without fear of this being revealed, that those owing duties of confidence in their employment should be loyal and should not disclose confidential matters and that, *prima facie*, no one should be allowed to use information extracted in breach of confidence from hospital records even if disclosure of the particular information may not give rise to immediately apparent harm. (p. 660)

Recognising the importance of the freedom of the press and that the nature of the information was such that there was some public interest in knowing about it he went on to stress:

> in my judgment those public interests are substantially outweighed when measured against the public interests in relation to loyalty and confidentiality both generally and with particular reference to AIDS patients' hospital records . . . victims of the disease ought not to be deterred by fear of discovery from going to hospital for treatment, and free and informed public debate about AIDS could take place without publication of the confidential information acquired by the defendants. (p. 661)

The judge in *X* v. *Y* concluded that the prevailing public interest should be to protect public health at large. If persons with HIV refuse testing and counselling because they fear that their confidences will not be kept, they are hurting themselves by not receiving the proper care and counselling and may therefore also become a threat to other people, by not appreciating how best to minimise the risk to others.

How helpful is the judgment in *X* v. *Y* in attempting to resolve the dispute about whether Carol's HIV status should be disclosed to her partner against her will? The facts of the two cases are very different. First, the disclosure in *X* v. *Y* was to the public at large, the vast majority of whom probably had a predominantly prurient interest in the subject. Second, the judge took careful account of evidence that in 1988 there was no recorded case of a health professional transmitting HIV to a patient and that the doctors in question were general practitioners unlikely to have any direct blood to blood contact with a patient. It is, in fact, the second of the court cases on medical confidentiality that gives us rather fuller guidance as to how the law approaches a breach of confidence committed to safeguard the health or safety of third parties.

In *W v. Egdell* (1989), W had been convicted of the manslaughter of five people. He had wounded two others and during the course of these events used hand-made explosives. At his trial he was diagnosed as suffering from schizophrenia and was detained as a patient in a secure hospital without time limit. Ten years after his detention he applied to a mental health review tribunal to be discharged or transferred to a regional secure unit with the ultimate aim of being discharged conditionally. W's consultant psychiatrist, Dr Ghosh, considered that W was cured of his illness and was no longer a threat to the public provided he received the appropriate medication. Dr Egdell was instructed by W's solicitors to examine W so that the report, which would follow, could be used to support W's application to the tribunal. Dr Egdell disagreed with Dr Ghosh's findings and suggested that W might be suffering from paranoid psychosis in which case medication would be less effective in preventing a relapse. He also intimated that W's illness might be due to a psychopathic deviant personality.

Unsurprisingly W's solicitors withdrew the application owing to the report to the tribunal, hoping no doubt to obtain a more favourable psychiatric opinion on a subsequent occasion. When Dr Egdell discovered this he contacted the medical director of the hospital, Dr Hunter. Dr Hunter finally agreed that the hospital should have a copy of the report in the interests of W's further treatment. A copy was sent to the hospital and then forwarded to the Home Secretary, who had the ultimate say as to whether and when W should ever be released from hospital.

W sued Dr Egdell, the hospital, the Home Secretary, and others for breach of the duty of confidence arising out of his relationship with Dr Egdell. His action failed. The trial judge said Dr Egdell did owe W a duty of confidence. He would, for example, have acted unlawfully if he had given W's story to the *Sun*. But in disclosing his findings to the hospital and the Home Secretary he acted lawfully.

> In my opinion, the duty he owed to W was not his only duty. W was not an ordinary member of the public . . . Dr Edgell owes a duty not only to his patient but also a duty to the public. His duty to the public would require him, in my opinion, to place before the proper authorities the result of his examination if, in his opinion, the public interest so required it. (p. 104)

Mr Justice Scott hence concluded that W presented a threat to the public and therefore it was in the interests of the public that Dr Egdell should breach his duty of confidence.

W went to the Court of Appeal but the appellate judges upheld the original findings of Mr Justice Scott. They stressed the public interest in medical confidentiality and emphasised that this applied as much to patients with mental illness, detained or otherwise, as to you or me. But in this case Lord Justice Bingham said:

> Where a man has committed multiple killings under the disability of serious mental illness, decisions which may lead directly or indirectly to his release from hospital should not be made unless the responsible authority is properly able to make an informed judgment that the risk of repetition is so small as to be acceptable. A consultant psychiatrist who becomes aware, even in the course of a confidential relationship, of information which leads him, in the exercise of what the court considers a sound professional judgment, to fear that such decisions may be made on inadequate information and with a real risk of consequent danger to the public is entitled to take such steps as are reasonable in all the circumstances to communicate the grounds of his concern to the responsible authorities. (p. 852)

The individual patient's right to confidentiality and the public interest in confidentiality, designed to ensure access to effective health care, are outweighed only where there is a real risk of harm or danger to others which can be averted by a breach of confidence. So if Pamela cannot persuade George to tell his employers of his epilepsy and cease to drive a fire engine, she may well be justified in contacting the DVLC. Just as W posed a risk of harm to others if released, so does George to other road users. Carol's HIV status is highly confidential. There could, for example, be no justification for telling her mum, however 'interested' her mum might be. Nor, for example, if Carol works as a teacher could you excuse informing her employers. But unless she can convince you otherwise, her partner is at risk. After all, as she is pregnant they must have had unprotected intercourse at least once. The difference between Carol on the one hand, and George and W on the other, is that she endangers only one other person. Is that difference relevant?

One final question must be addressed. In our discussion of ethical considerations it was argued that there might be cases where it was not only justifiable to breach confidence, there was a moral imperative to do so. And we saw that an American court in the Tarasoff case found that a failure to warn Tatiana and her family of the risk posed to her rendered the University of California liable for her death. Such a mandatory duty to break confidence has never been imposed by an English court as yet. And currently the English courts are reluctant to hold X liable for a wrong actually committed by Y unless X has an actual duty to control Y's behaviour, for example, Y is a prisoner in custody. The most tricky situation is where both the individual to whom you owe the duty of confidentiality and the person at risk are your patients. You have a direct duty to both of them, as does the practice nurse in Carol's case.

Your colleagues' confidences – whistleblowing

Report to an appropriate person or authority, having regard to the physical, psychological and social effects on patients and clients, any circumstances in the environment of care which could jeopardise standards of practice. (Clause eleven, *Code of Professional Conduct*)

Report to an appropriate person or authority any circumstance in which safe and appropriate care for patients and clients cannot be provided. (Clause twelve, *Code of Professional Conduct*)

Your patients are not the only people who will impart confidences to you. Your colleagues will too. Your employer will entrust you with sensitive information which in a competitive NHS could be harmful to your hospital if released. Normally, of course, you should preserve such confidences just as you protect a patient's confidences. If nothing else, common sense and courtesy suggest you do not tell Dr Smith that Sister White thinks he is overweight and 'past it'! Today, though, there is increasing concern that doctors and nurses put protecting each other, and each other's confidences, above the welfare of their patients. If by 'past it' Sister White means Dr Smith can no longer do his job, do you have a duty to act? Hospitals increasingly try to impose confidentiality on their staff. If you are a research nurse working on a potentially profitable new drug it is reasonable (and lawful) to stop you trying to sell the formula to a rival. But what if you believe the hospital's operating theatres are unsafe because of cutbacks on cleaning? Can you, should you, act even if that means breaching confidence with your employer and your colleagues? In 1994, in the wake of several scandals, 'whistleblowing' is as much of a crucial issue as preserving patients' confidences. A whistleblower is someone who, having discovered a practice within the workplace which could be considered negligent or harmful, decides to draw attention to it. The information is often offered to the public at large, and given to an outside body such as a pressure group or a newspaper as perhaps attempts to remedy matters internally have failed. Sometimes the whistleblower chooses to leak information anonymously and, although this is likely to be less effective than information backed by an identifiable individual, anonymity does afford some protection to the person leaking the information. For the practical problem that whistleblowers encounter, however justifiable their action, is how to make the public aware of negligent or harmful practices without jeopardising their own careers. In practice this appears extremely difficult to do as the recent real-life case involving Graham Pink demonstrates. Mr Pink faced a stark conflict between his duty of loyalty to his employers and his professional responsibilities to protect the welfare of his patients.

The Pink case

Graham Pink was a night charge nurse at Stepping Hill Hospital, Stockport, who, along with another charge nurse, was responsible for a unit consisting of three wards. One ward had twenty beds and the other two twenty-six beds each. Only patients over seventy-five years of age are admitted to these wards. The patients suffered from a variety of illnesses such as arthritis, diabetes, congestive cardiac failure or had experienced a cerebro-vascular accident, as well as many of the disabilities of the elderly, such as confusion, incontinence, deafness, poor eyesight and immobility. The nursing staff allocation for the three wards at night was alleged to be as follows: for the twenty-six-bedded ward, one trained and two untrained nurses, for each of the twenty-bedded wards, one trained and one untrained nurse to cover an eleven-hour period.

Mr Pink, a local magistrate as well as an experienced nurse, considered that staffing levels were totally inadequate and, having tried and failed to win any support from within the nursing management in the hospital, he wrote almost 100 letters to various people including the chairman of the health authority, consultant geriatricians, the UKCC, MPs, the Department of Health and the Prime Minister, in an attempt to alert them to the danger the patients were in because of poor staffing. Ultimately he contacted the media and his complaints received extensive media attention including articles in *The Guardian* and the *Nursing Times*, which commissioned an expert in quality assurance to assess the staffing levels in the unit. Mr Pink and the relevant journalists took care to safeguard the dignity and privacy of individual patients.

On 9 August 1990, Mr Pink was called to a disciplinary meeting where he was suspended from duty on allegations of breaching confidentiality and making an error in drug administration. Stockport Health Authority issued a twenty-two page statement regarding the system used to determine staffing levels and alleged that Mr Pink's actions had damaged public confidence in the hospital and staff morale and had breached patient confidences. In November 1990, following a lengthy disciplinary hearing, managers at Stockport Health Authority found him guilty of gross misconduct. He was then offered a community nursing post as an alternative to dismissal.

Mr Pink proved a doughty opponent. He had come back to nursing late in life and had a pension earned from another career. He rejected the health authority's 'punishment' and took his case to an industrial tribunal complaining of unfair dismissal. Three years later the authority backed down half-way through the tribunal hearing and at least partially conceded Mr Pink's case that they had acted unfairly towards him, although they continued to reject his allegations about unsatisfactory patient care. But how many nurses have the resources, human or financial, to fight the kind of lonely battle Graham Pink faced?

Despite media coverage and support from the UKCC, RCN and other trade unions, and his ultimate success, the result of his actions will inevitably operate as a deterrent for other nurses wanting to expose negligent or harmful practices in the workplace. As a charge nurse, Mr Pink was responsible for the delivery of care to patients on the unit of which he was in charge during his span of duty. If he was not able to ensure that the delivery of this care was to acceptable standards, then to fail to inform the relevant people of this fact would have been contrary to his professional code of ethics, clauses eleven and twelve of the *Code of Professional Conduct*. Yet disciplinary hearings are controlled by the very health authority or NHS trust against whom allegations are made, and the actual individuals with whom the whistleblower has been in dispute may be on the panel made up for the disciplinary hearing. Support may be given by the UKCC and trade unions, but there are no practical means by which they can protect a nurse from a health authority disciplinary hearing with a biased panel. Nurses are faced with a dilemma: if they speak out about what they consider poor standards of care they may face disciplinary action by their employers, and if they remain silent, they are breaching the *Code of Professional Conduct* and are liable to disciplinary action from the UKCC. This situation has been further complicated by the inclusion of so-called 'gagging' clauses in contracts of employment by some NHS trusts seeking to prevent health professionals drawing poor standards to the attention of the public. Whistleblowers may all too often find that they are accused of disregarding loyalty to colleagues by reporting either within or outside the workplace practices considered to be negligent or harmful. Where does the proper balance between loyalty to patients and colleagues lie? Think about the following case studies.

The concerned student

Antony Black is a student nurse currently gaining experience on a care of the elderly ward as part of the Project 2000 course. He has become concerned about the attitudes of some of the trained staff towards the patients in ward three, the long-term care ward. Many of these patients have been resident in the hospital for a long period of time, and Antony feels that they are treated with little respect or dignity.

Antony discusses his concerns with the other student nurses taking the same module and he discovers that they share his reservations about the care that patients receive. He volunteers to speak to the tutor responsible for the Care of the Elderly module about the situation on ward three, and to request that action be taken about the care these patients receive.

The following day, Antony is approached by Ann, one of the student nurses who had joined in the discussion about ward three the previous day. She tells him that he is unlikely to get any support from the other student nurses if he speaks to the tutor about the ward. She explains that she knows that a student complained the year previously, but the student was accused of being disloyal to colleagues by the staff on ward three and experienced difficulties during the assessment of her clinical competence as a consequence. Ann reminds Antony that they are approaching the end of their course and that jobs in the hospital are in short supply. She says that most of the students are worried about the job situation and feel that speaking out in this way might count against them.

Antony realises that faced with no support from the other students his claims might not be so effective. He is also worried about job opportunities and so decides to remain silent.

The unseen examination

Susan Huxley is a registered nurse working on a gynaecological ward in a large university teaching hospital. The education of students is an important part of the hospital's work and all patients are aware that students may be involved in their care. Although patients have the right to refuse to allow students to participate in their care, it is up to the individual concerned to lodge her objection as it is assumed that there are no objections to this practice, unless specified. As Susan has spent a very small amount of time in the operating theatre in the past, she decides that it would be beneficial for her to be present in theatre one day to observe surgery. Susan expressly chooses to watch Mr Fielding operate as she is aware that he is considered to be an excellent teacher.

The following week, Susan arrives in the operating theatre to watch Mr Fielding. The patient is anaesthetised and then brought into the theatre. Mr Fielding explains the procedure to three medical students who are also observing and then suggests that they each perform a vaginal examination on the woman to practise this procedure. Susan is unhappy about this and asks one of the theatre sisters if this is common practice. The sister tells her that Mr Fielding always lets students practise vaginal examinations on women when they are anaesthetised.

During the course of the day, Susan has an opportunity to ask Mr Fielding about this practice. He responds by saying that the students have to learn and that it is not harmful to the women because they are anaesthetised and so unaware of what is happening. Susan asks if the women are informed about this and if their consent is obtained, but Mr Fielding tells her that it is not necessary to trouble the women with information of this sort especially as they are probably already anxious about surgery and the examination does no harm. Mr Fielding stresses the importance of the educational role the hospital fulfils and reminds her that patients have the right to refuse to have students participating in their care and can make members of staff aware of this. Susan is unhappy about his explanation and believes that the women have no idea what is being done to them. Susan decides that women should be alerted to what is going on so that they can refuse to allow this sort of examination. She contacts a journalist on the local newspaper and asks her to write an article exposing this practice.

Loyalty to colleagues

Because a whistleblower comes from within an organisation, to disclose information about colleagues can cause accusations of disloyalty to be made against the whistleblower. Although nurses make no particular promises or oaths of loyalty, because they work as part of a large team delivering health care, a certain amount of loyalty is naturally expected of them. Nurses thus can find themselves in situations where they know patient care is being compromised, but fear that to report this is betraying the confidences of a colleague who may well be a friend.

Suppose that Laura, a staff nurse in the intensive care unit knows that Sandra, another nurse in the same unit, has been drinking alcohol before coming on duty. Although Sandra may not appear to be actually drunk, working in an intensive care unit calls for a highly specialised form of nursing, and even small amounts of alcohol can make a person less observant and alert. Laura may be reluctant to tell the sister in charge of the unit about Sandra, particularly if Sandra has told her of her drinking in confidence. To resolve a situation like this a nurse must assess what actions are likely to cause the most harm, either to the patients, because of the risk of receiving care at less than acceptable standards, or to the colleague, by being reported and possibly facing disciplinary procedures. The nurse may feel that she has a duty to protect the interests of the patients and this is of overriding importance whatever the consequences to one's colleague.

The UKCC is clear as to how the nurse should act. The *Code of Professional Conduct* clearly states that the interests of patients must predominate over those of practitioner and profession, and would therefore expect any nurse finding themselves in Laura's position to protect the interests of the patients. But the position is not always as simple as this in practice as discussion of the case studies involving Antony and Susan will demonstrate.

Antony Black, the student, was faced with a conflict of interests, the interests of the patients and self-interest. Antony has to decide which interests are of more importance and act accordingly. If he decides that the interests of the patients are more important, then he is acting ethically in accordance with clause eleven of the *Code of Professional Conduct*. He would be justified in making complaints about the staff on the ward in question. If he decides his own interests are of more importance, then he will need to find other reasons to support this claim. One such reason might be that it is better to effect change from within, and that perhaps if Antony says nothing on this occasion, but waits until he is a qualified nurse then he may be able to bring about changes in patient care, especially if he actively seeks a post on this ward. By arguing in this way, Antony might still claim that he was acting in the interests of the patients, as his aim is to bring about a change in patient care rather than ensure that he is given a job at the end of his training. Or would he simply be placating his own conscience?

The issues in Susan's case are very different. To blow the whistle effectively, Susan must be sure of the facts of the case. It would appear that Susan has not only witnessed what is happening but also discussed Mr Fielding's reasons for allowing the examinations to take place. It is also important to decide if the information, even if it is accurate, is information which the general public is entitled to know, or in this case, private information that only members of staff need know. Susan may argue that this is information which it is in the interests of the public to know, and that women should be given an opportunity to refuse to allow such an examination to be performed. Mr Fielding could argue that if women refused, the students' education would suffer and this is more important, especially as the women are not being harmed. Of course, what is important here is what constitutes harming the patient, and whether this is restricted to actual physical harm.

The third issue is to do with whom the whistleblower tells. Susan decides to say nothing more about the case, but go directly to the press. She obviously feels strongly that this method of treatment is wrong. However, it may be argued that she should have made her objections known to the theatre sister, manager or Mr Fielding himself before reporting the case to an outside body. If she had still received no satisfactory explanation from them, only then would she be justified in 'going public'. This was the course of action adopted by Graham Pink who attempted to alert his own nurse managers and the health authority to the poor staffing levels on his wards before resorting to outside bodies.

Susan needs to assess in whose interests she is acting. Even though she is acting in the interests of her patients, Susan should be sure that she has acted in the most effective way to bring about change.

Whistleblowers and the law

The law will on occasion protect confidences imparted between friends and colleagues as well as those deriving from professional relationships. So in *Stephens* v. *Avery* (1988) a 'false friend' was banned from selling an account confided to her of a lesbian love affair. If a colleague confides in you that she has been sleeping with a married charge nurse, it may be unlawful as well as disloyal to breach her confidence.

Undoubtedly the nurse, like any other employee, owes a duty of fidelity to her employer, and this includes a duty to keep confidences and so not damage the employer's 'business'. That duty exists whether or not there is any express 'gagging clause' in the contract of employment. Unjustifiable disclosure of your employer's confidences is unlawful. But note that word 'unjustifiable'. Just as the law will excuse a breach of patient confidentiality if disclosure is justified in the public interest, so the law sanctions breach of employers' confidences where other factors outweigh the nurse's duty to her employer. Evidence of criminal conduct is an obvious example of justifiable disclosure. But in *Lion Laboratories Ltd* v. *Evans* (1984) the Court of Appeal held that whenever harm to the public might ensue and all other methods to avert that harm had failed, the employee was justified in breaching confidence. In that case the employee had evidence that the design of breathalyser made by the firm that he worked for was defective. He told his employers who took no action. His ultimate disclosure to the press was found to be justified.

In theory, the genuine whistleblower has little to fear from the law relating to employee confidentiality. First, the law only protects truly confidential information. It does not create a duty to remain silent on all matters relating to your job or the practice of your profession. Antony is not legally prohibited from criticising his colleagues. In the Graham Pink case much of what Mr Pink described was public knowledge. Information gleaned from patient and staff records is confidential, and results of audit and discussion on practice all may well be confidential too. Second, even where the information in question is truly confidential, if a practice or behaviour is endangering patient care, disclosure will be lawful and justified by virtue of the public interest defence. In the first instance disclosure should be as limited as possible. Antony is right to seek first to express his concerns to his course tutor. Susan should not go to the press without first seeking to remedy her complaints with the hospital and professional authorities. But if all else fails, public disclosure can be justified to remedy real failures in the service.

Practice is more problematic. If you breach confidence with your employer, then just like an aggrieved patient he could go to court and sue you for damages or ask for an injunction preventing you repeating that breach of confidence. That way you at least get your day in court and the chance to put your side of the story. Alas, what your employer is more likely to do is, as in the Graham Pink case, to try to discipline you or even sack you.

Another practical example of the difficulties whistleblowers face can be seen in the case of *Callanan* v. *Surrey Area Health Authority* (1980). Callanan was a student nurse at a psychiatric hospital. He and another student nurse had seen a charge nurse hitting patients and administering drug overdoses. He wrote a confidential letter to the hospital's nursing officer who passed it on to a senior nursing officer. When investigations were initiated the nurse whom Callanan had accused, along with others, threatened to stop work if Callanan and another nurse reported for duty on the wards. The report written after the investigation did not comment on whether the allegations were correct but stated that the allegations had been made in good faith and there was no reason why Callanan and the other nurse should not return to work. Industrial problems followed the incident and Callanan was expelled from COHSE, his union. Management then told him that he would only be allowed to return to work if he acknowledged that his allegations were inaccurate. If he failed to do so, the period in which he had been absent from the ward because of the incident would not be counted as training time. He resigned and alleged that the health authority's actions amounted to constructive dismissal – in that he had no choice but to resign. His claim was upheld by an industrial tribunal which held that his dismissal had not been justified. Even though the industrial tribunal upheld his claim he was not reinstated although he did receive some compensation. It is important that Callanan's disclosure was limited to hospital management. A nurse who went straight to the press, without trying to redress grievances locally first, would probably not be vindicated by a tribunal.

Proposals and guidance

As is very obvious, the major dilemma in whistleblowing is that even if the whistleblower is morally and legally justified in what she does, she may still suffer from being right. In 1992 the RCN put forward an agenda for reform of whistleblowing. The first proposal was that each unit should establish an agreed protocol for expressing concerns about patient care, and staff who invoked the protocol would be able to do so without fear of reprisal. Further, they recommended that the UKCC *Code of Professional Conduct* should be incorporated into employment contracts. Some authorities already do this. However, as you have seen, the code itself provides conflicting duties where confidential information is concerned. The RCN demanded that express 'gagging' clauses should be abolished, and access to counselling should be available for nurses under pressure at work. The Government should set agreed standards of care for each service, providing an objective standard setting procedure and a national inspectorate for health care should be established. Finally, legislative protection should be provided for the whistleblower.

The Department of Health issued draft guidelines on the question of whistleblowing in October 1992. The guidelines provide that NHS line managers have an obligation to ensure that all staff feel that they are able to express their concerns and that such complaints will be fairly and sympathetically considered. Complaint procedures, it is recommended, should be drawn up locally and as long as employees raise complaints in good faith they should not be penalised. The purpose is to enable matters to be resolved informally between the individual and the line manager. If it is considered inappropriate or impractical to take up a complaint, the complainant must be given a thorough explanation. If the complainant is not satisfied he or she should be able to refer the complaint up the management structure ultimately to the chairman of the health authority or trust. An alternative route is also suggested – that a senior officer be appointed to receive complaints from patients under the Hospital Complaints Procedures.

The reforms may not lessen the burden on nurses and other health professionals – complaints must still be made within the system, existing fears are therefore not removed. If local action fails, what does the nurse do? Can she be expected to act to protect patients at the risk of her own career?

Subject access – the patient's right to know

One final issue relating to confidentiality must be addressed. The most sensitive confidential information entrusted to nurses obviously relates to their patients. To whom does that information belong – is it the 'property' of the professional or the patient? Traditionally doctors have tended to regard that information as 'theirs'. This had two consequences. While doctors recognised their legal and ethical obligation not to disclose their patients' secrets to unrelated third parties, they felt free to share that information with other members of the health care team and on occasion with the patient's family. And very often they withheld information from patients themselves, considering the patient was better left in ignorance. Who does have the right of access to information recorded in patients' notes? The patient gives a nurse confidential information which is then written in the patient's records, but many other people such as physiotherapists, dieticians, radiographers, and even ward clerks will then have access to this information which may be seen by the patient as a breach of confidentiality, should they be aware of it. One study carried out in

America indicated that as many as seventy-five people involved in some way with the care of the patient had access to patients' records.

Health professionals very frequently share confidential information about a patient amongst themselves without the patient's knowledge. This may be used to discuss methods of treatment or aspects of nursing care, or present case studies. There are situations in clinical practice, particularly when a terminal illness has been diagnosed, when the diagnosis is discussed first with the next of kin, relatives or even friends of the patient before the patient is informed. It is not uncommon following such a discussion for it to be decided that the patient should not be informed of the diagnosis, so that several people then share confidential information about a patient that he remains totally unaware of.

In this sort of situation, it may be argued that the health professional withholding the information from the patient is acting in the patient's interests and according to the principle of non-maleficence. Although this may be true, it may not be what the patient wants, and it can prove difficult to decide which is the best course of action to follow. One solution is to allow patients access to their medical records. If the patient wanted to know more about their illness including the diagnosis and prognosis, then a request to look at their records would indicate to health professionals that the patient wanted more information, and that withholding such information might be inappropriate in this case.

Before the Access to Health Records Act 1990 a patient had no legal right of access to information or records held about him in manual files. The Data Protection Act 1984 had given patients a limited right of access to computerised files. The only information that a nurse was obliged to give was that information which it was necessary and reasonable to give, in order to ensure that the patient received adequate health care. The nurse has a duty to disclose to the patient those risks which it is normal nursing practice to disclose. She need not disclose every detail if it is not necessary for adequate treatment, or for the patient to give an effective consent to treatment. The conservative approach of the English judiciary to 'informed consent' was discussed in the previous chapter.

The Access to Health Records Act now provides that where a record made by or on behalf of a health professional contains 'information about the physical or mental health of an identifiable individual', that individual has a right of access to the relevant information. A patient who wants access must apply in writing to the record holder (generally either the GP, health authority or NHS trust) and is entitled both to access to the record and to an explanation if information is not intelligible. If the record holder decides that certain parts of the record may cause serious physical or mental harm to the patient or another individual, he or she may refuse access to those parts of the record. Access may also be refused if the holder believes that disclosure could lead to the identification of someone other than the patient or of a health professional involved in the care of the patient. The Act applies only to records compiled after November 1991.

The patient's right of access is quite easily curtailed – if he is unaware that crucial information has been withheld he will not know that he could have a remedy in court. Even if he is told that information has been kept back, the court simply reviews the record holder's decision and if it agrees with the decision to withhold, the patient still has no access and no right to compensation.

6

Justice and the allocation of resources

Recognise and respect the uniqueness and dignity of each patient and client, and respond to their need for care, religious beliefs, personal attributes, the nature of their health problems or any other factor. (Clause seven, *Code of Professional Conduct*)

Justice

The principles of justice can be explained in different ways. One of the most simple ways is perhaps the Aristotelian view that equals should be treated equally and unequals treated unequally. Justice can also be understood in terms of what people deserve, either as rewards or punishments, and an example of this would be giving prison sentences or fines to people convicted of criminal offences. We might also say that a person who fulfilled all the criteria necessary for becoming a registered nurse should be given this status and it would be an unjust action to deprive this person of registration. Alternatively, justice can be understood in terms of fairness whereby a person's claim to something is based upon a morally relevant property such as need.

Within the concept of justice as a whole, you can make a distinction between distributive justice and corrective justice. Distributive justice is concerned with the distribution of goods within society, whereas corrective justice is concerned with punishments that may be made for offences committed within society. The issues raised in this chapter about the allocation of health care resources are concerned with distributive rather than corrective justice.

Problems of distributive justice only occur when there is a shortage of goods within society. If, for example, it was possible to provide every person who needed it with renal dialysis, then many of the difficult questions about whom to treat would simply not arise. Of course it may be suggested that not everyone who needs access to health care facilities deserves to be treated; what about people who require surgery for a smoking-related illness? Although our discussion concerns access to health care, remember that the same problems occur in any society where there are shortages of goods or services. They are of crucial importance when basics such as food or clean water are scarce.

Two further distinctions must be made, between macro-allocation and micro-allocation of resources. Decisions about resource allocation that take place at a macro level are about the amount of funds allocated to health care by the government as well as decisions about the amount of funding that should be given to differing specialities such as paediatrics, obstetrics, psychiatry, or care of the elderly. There is an ethical dimension to this decision-making process because difficult decisions have to be made, between specialities if there is insufficient funding available, and on whether services such as infertility treatments should be funded at all. Micro-allocation of resources is concerned with deciding which individuals actually receive the resources allocated. These decisions may be about the priority in which patients are admitted to hospital, or treated in an accident and emergency department, or they may concern which patients should be treated at all if resources are inadequate.

The allocation of medical resources has become an increasingly important subject discussed not only by those directly concerned with the provision of health services but, because of its implications, amongst many differing sections of society. Improvement in medical, surgical and diagnostic services as well as new pharmacological discoveries has meant that conditions once thought impossible to treat effectively can now be more easily diagnosed and treated. In the United Kingdom where health care services are provided by the State, it has become obvious that it is impossible for all forms of treatment to be available to every person who may require them, and in some cases patients may have to be denied treatment. This has resulted in conflict between what health professionals want and perhaps feel they ought to provide, and what patients need and perhaps have a right to expect should be provided. The following case studies illustrate these sorts of conflicts.

The child with a severe disability

Mr and Mrs Yates have one child, Ben, aged ten, who is severely physically and mentally disabled, as a result of cerebral palsy. Ben cannot sit upright unless supported by a special chair, and is totally dependent upon his parents for all basic human needs. Ben is unable to talk, and gives no indication that he understands anything that has been said to him. However, Mrs Yates maintains that they have developed their own system of communication over the years. Ben is cared for at home by his parents with some assistance from social services. Mr and Mrs Yates have made many sacrifices because of their child, but they consider it their parental responsibility and provide a very caring home for Ben to live in. Occasionally Ben is admitted to a children's ward at the local hospital to allow Mr and Mrs Yates a holiday.

During his current admission to the hospital, Ben has developed a chest infection. The infection has not responded to antibiotic treatment and Ben's condition is deteriorating. The paediatrician has suggested that the only course of action is to admit Ben to the intensive care unit so that he can be given mechanical ventilation to stabilise his condition. But there is only one empty bed in the intensive care unit. Dr Nelson, the consultant in charge of the unit, has objected to Ben being admitted to this bed. He argues that there are patients undergoing major surgery in the hospital that day who may need intensive care facilities following surgery. He thinks that there are more urgent cases than Ben when resources are scarce, and that it would be much kinder just to let 'nature take its course' when a child has such a poor quality of life.

The dying AIDS patient

St Luke's is a hospice managed by Roman Catholic nuns which has built up an excellent local reputation for terminal care. The hospital is registered as a charity and relies on fund-raising initiatives from the local community for its continued existence.

Recently a request has been made by a general practitioner to admit one of her patients, Peter, a young man dying from AIDS. Initially Peter's family cared for him at home but the deterioration in his condition has now made it impossible to continue to do so. Peter's family has requested that he be admitted to St Luke's. They feel sure that he will be able to spend the remainder of his life in comfort there. This is the first time a request has been made to admit a patient suffering from AIDS. Dr Wall, the physician in charge, agrees to admit Peter to the hospice.

Sister Dunne has worked at the hospice since it opened eight years ago. As well as being employed full-time as a nurse, she devotes much time and energy to fund-raising activities for the hospice. She objects to Dr Wall's decision to admit patients suffering from AIDS and asks that the matter be referred to the hospital management committee. Dr Wall and Sister Dunne are invited to put forward their views.

Dr Wall suggests that the hospice exists to provide terminal care to any patient that requires it, and therefore there are no grounds to discriminate against an AIDS sufferer. Sister Dunne argues that admitting a patient with AIDS would damage public relations, as she feels that many members of the general public would be afraid of entering a hospice which cared for AIDS patients because of risk of infection. She is particularly concerned about the number of voluntary workers who help in the running of the hospice. In addition, Sister Dunne fears that financial support might also be lost.

The management committee see that both arguments are relevant, but ultimately want to come to a decision that will not damage the high esteem in which the hospice is held. The committee members realise that either rejecting or accepting patients suffering from AIDS is likely to be controversial and find it difficult to decide on the best course of action.

Justice and equality

Treating people as equals

All people who come into contact with health care services should expect to be treated on an equal basis both because they have a common need, and because as citizens they are equally entitled to the care and protection of the State as expressed in its public institutions like the provision of health care. Society obviously would not tolerate the setting up of a hospital that would only treat white men under the age of sixty.

Dworkin in *Taking Rights Seriously* has shown that there are two rather different considerations when talking about equality: firstly, the claim that individuals have to equal treatment, and secondly, the different claim that an individual has to be treated as an equal. A claim to equal treatment is the claim to an equal distribution of a resource within society such as each citizen in a democracy has to one vote or that someone has to a hospital bed when necessary. Although there are differences between people such as their race, gender, height or employment, these differences are not significant when resources like votes or hospital beds are to be distributed amongst the members of a society. Very few people would suggest that someone who was employed should be entitled to more than one vote or those unemployed should be denied a vote. Equality therefore is not a descriptive term that we can apply to individuals in the same way as race or gender.

Suppose that I belong to the St John Ambulance Brigade, and one Saturday afternoon I am on duty at a football match when an accident occurs resulting in several casualties to whom I have to administer first aid. As it is impossible for me to treat everyone at the same time, the first question that I may ask myself is how to decide whom to treat first, as all the injured people have a claim to equal treatment. It would not make sense for me to select one group of people to treat, without being able to justify why I have selected that particular group over another. I may decide to treat only women and justify this by saying that they may have young children at home dependent on them. Although this may be true, the only conclusions I can draw about this group is that they are all women, but this fact alone does not enable me to make assumptions about the number of dependent children each one may have. Not all women in the crowd may have dependent children and there may be several men who do, whom I would be more justified in treating than childless women.

I may choose to treat any children first and justify that decision by saying that they have the rest of their lives before them and deserve to be given a chance to live. Again, perhaps some of the children are terminally ill and may be expected to die soon anyway no matter what sort of treatment I may give them. Although small children will obviously be candidates for immediate treatment using this scheme, I may find it less easy to differentiate between a child and a young adult. No matter which group I may select to treat first, it is difficult to make general statements about all women, all children, all men or all people of a particular race that will hold true for every individual within that group. Although we can acknowledge that there are differences between individuals, knowledge of some differences does not as a result allow us to infer other facts about a person. So for the purposes of access to health care facilities, it should be possible to disregard broad divisions such as race or sex and treat all patients as equals.

The implications of equality

Although it may appear that to disregard broad divisions amongst people and treat all patients as equals is the right way for health professionals to operate, there are other factors to take into consideration. As well as recognising the claim that individuals have to equal treatment, a second claim is recognised, that is, the claim that people have to be treated as equals. This is different from claiming a right to equal treatment as it suggests that any person should expect to be treated with the same respect as any other person, irrespective of any differences between them.

Returning to the same accident at the football match, suppose that I have been convinced of the necessity to give all the injured people equal treatment. As I steadily work my way through the injured people in the crowd, I come across two people lying side by side, one of whom has a fractured arm, and the other who is bleeding severely from a wound. By this time I only have two bandages left in my first aid box and I know that to treat these people equally I should give them one bandage each. However, I also know that although one bandage is enough to support the injured arm and make that person comfortable, I will need both bandages to stand any chance of stopping the bleeding from the wound on the other person. If I give two bandages to one person then I have none to give to the other and so I am not treating them equally, but the person with the bleeding wound may die if I cannot stop the bleeding, whereas the person with the fractured arm will be in pain, but is not likely to die.

If I give each victim one bandage each, although I could not be accused of giving these people unequal treatment, it could be argued that I am not recognising a claim to treatment as an equal, that is, the right that each of them has to be treated with the same respect as the other. If I give each of them a bandage, then although I am alleviating the pain of the person with the fractured arm, I am endangering the life of the person with the bleeding wound, so I have not demonstrated equal concern. There are two undesirable outcomes to consider here: firstly, that the person with the fractured arm will be in pain if I do not give him one of the bandages, and, secondly, that the person with the bleeding wound is likely to die if I do not give him both bandages.

As a person giving first aid, I should avoid endangering life, and so if I want to show equal respect and concern for both these two injured people, I must give the person with the bleeding wound both bandages and leave the person with the fractured arm without a bandage. To do otherwise is to say that the life of the person with the bleeding wound counts for nothing in comparison to alleviating the pain of the other injured person, and that it is therefore permissible to allow that person to die in order to make the other more comfortable. People, despite their differences, have equal moral importance and therefore have equal dependence upon each other and the State.

This is, of course, the way that health services usually operate. For example, patients are seen in a casualty department according to the order in which they arrive, but seriously ill people such as victims of road traffic accidents or someone suffering a myocardial infarction are treated immediately. Similarly, most hospitals have waiting lists for people requiring surgery, but a person requiring surgery for coronary artery disease or for cancer will be given priority over those requiring surgery for less serious illnesses. It seems then, that people are not treated equally and that all do not have equal access to health care but that some system of priority operates.

In general people do not seem to object to this sort of prioritisation as it would be unlikely that someone waiting in a casualty department with a minor injury would insist on being seen before someone seriously injured simply because they had been waiting longer. If someone did raise an objection of this sort there would probably be little sympathy for this point of view from others. The only way people could be treated equally in hospital would be if there was always at least one doctor, one nurse and one bed available for every patient as well as enough equipment and personnel for immediate access to diagnostic services, which is, alas, impossible. Why are people prepared to be treated in an unequal manner without question in these situations? One answer is that most of us do have a sense of urgency regarding differing medical situations and are able automatically to prioritise cases ourselves. Alternatively, people may be prepared to be treated unequally in this way out of self-interest. Because every person has the potential to be the seriously injured casualty requiring immediate treatment, if such an event occurred, this person would then probably want to be treated as a priority.

This type of consideration and decision-making process is undertaken by people involved with health care at all levels within society. It is undertaken at a macro level by those in Government making decisions about how much to spend on health as opposed to education or defence, by health authorities about how much to spend on maternity services as opposed to the mentally ill or the elderly, by hospital managers about whether to cut surgical waiting lists by using day surgery facilities, but cause ward closures and staff redundancies as a result. It happens at a micro level at the start of the day when a staff nurse decides which of the five patients allocated to her care she should see first. It is a necessary process because it is impossible to treat all people requiring health care services on an equal basis, unless each and every one of us has our own exclusive health care team constantly on duty.

Allocation of resources

Earlier in this chapter we suggested that all individuals should have equal access to health care facilities and that it is difficult to justify denying people this on the grounds of broad divisions within society such as sex or race. To deny someone treatment because they are black or male is unacceptable because it would count as unjust discrimination. Society appears to accept the fact that priority in health care services should be given to those most in need and this, as a result, should cut across all of the broad divisions that exist within our society. Unfortunately the situation in real life is far more complex than this as resources may still be inadequate for patients who undoubtably need priority treatment on clinical grounds, causing other difficult decisions to be made about whom to treat.

Even if broad divisions such as sex or race are disregarded as grounds for deciding how to allocate health services, there are other types of differences between individuals that have to be considered. Some may argue that the only fair way to allocate resources is to treat people at random, others argue that it is better to treat those in greatest clinical need. You could aim to treat the greatest number of people, or treat the young rather than the elderly, or treat able-bodied people rather than the disabled, or those who have become ill due to no fault of their own rather than those who have become ill due to their own actions such as smokers or heroin addicts. The issues are further complicated if you take into consideration how resources are allocated at a higher level. Should teaching hospitals have more funds than non-teaching hospitals, or should the emphasis be on preventative medicine such as vaccination programmes, rather than curative medicine such as transplant surgery? Should mentally disabled people have institutional care or care in the community?

Treating people at random

One method of avoiding such questions is to disregard all information about people such as their age or the severity of their illness, and allocate resources entirely at random. In this way people who needed access to health care services would take part in some sort of lottery to decide who would receive treatment. Such a method might be attractive to health professionals because it takes away the need for a difficult decision to be made by one person or by a group of individuals about whom to treat. If there are six people waiting for admission to a hospital bed and there is only one bed available, then the bed could be allocated by pulling numbers out of a hat or running a computer programme to select at random the person to be admitted. In this way each patient has an equal chance of being admitted to hospital and no person is favoured over another.

Allocating resources at random may ensure that people have an equal chance at receiving treatment but such a system is unlikely to be accepted as a fair way of choosing whom to treat. Objections to this sort of lottery are that it is more just to treat those in need first, or children rather than the elderly. Yet it is not sufficient to say that it is more just to treat those in need first, without saying why such individuals should have priority access to limited resources. In other words, although this may be the right way to act, we should also be able to justify our actions by demonstrating why it is the right way to act.

Treating the first in line

If the idea of running a lottery to allocate medical resources is rejected because it leaves too much to chance, then the next sort of policy that may be considered is one that allows some sort of intervention but without discriminating between individuals.

Returning again to the accident at the football match, suppose I have been convinced of the necessity to treat all individuals as equals and set about giving first aid to those who are injured. I cannot treat more than one person at a time, so I may decide to start with the nearest injured person to me and then gradually work my way through the crowd. Although it is unlikely that anyone would accuse me of actively discriminating against certain individuals if I work in this way, the treatment I am giving could be largely ineffective. I may find that the people nearest to me had only minor injuries and I have used up all my first aid supplies on them and so have nothing left for the seriously injured person further away from me. Although I am undoubtably treating the injured people impartially, it could be argued that in doing so I am not treating them with equal respect and concern. People can be given equal treatment by distributing resources equally amongst them, but in order to treat people as equals, you must consider how the treatment will affect their respective dignity and standing as equal members of the community.

Treating those most in need

Perhaps a more attractive argument is to disregard all other factors about individuals apart from their clinical need for treatment. To return to the accident at the football match, I may now be convinced of the arguments to give people equal treatment, but also to treat them with equal respect and concern. Hence I reject the idea of treating those closest to me and decide to assess the injuries of the people in a given area and prioritise the cases, treating those in most need first. Working in this way I hope to distribute the first aid equipment I have with me and my skills by treating those most in need first. Suppose I assess twenty people and find that twelve of them have minor injuries and eight of them are seriously injured. I decide to treat the seriously injured first, but all eight people really need my urgent attention. I still cannot treat more than one patient at a time, so I still have to decide in what order I should treat them. Should I treat the children rather than the elderly, the men with families rather than the childless men, or the people usually healthy before the diabetics, those with heart disease or the physically disabled? I am also aware that if I treat those with minor injuries they will probably not need hospital admission but those seriously injured will, no matter what first aid treatment I can give them.

Suppose that despite my treatment all of the seriously injured people die, it might be argued that I have wasted my time and really should have been attending to the minor injuries first and as a result saved twelve people from needing more intensive treatment later on because of missing out on first aid treatment. There is a policy called triage that exists ostensibly to cope with the large number of casualties in times of war. Survivors are divided into three groups as follows:

1. Those who will die despite treatment.
2. Those who will live even without treatment.
3. Those whose survival depends upon being given treatment.

In time of war not only may there be a shortage of dressings and drugs, but also a shortage of time and staff with the necessary skills to treat all the casualties. As a result, only the casualties whose survival depends upon being given treatment will receive it.

Triage in its original context may be considered a harsh system to use, as decisions have to be made that some people should not be given any treatment at all, and therefore left to die, but this system has been modified for use in accident and emergency departments and is now commonly used. What happens in emergency units is that all patients are assessed on their arrival in the department by a triage nurse who decides the extent of each person's injuries, how urgently they need to be treated and by which member of the accident and emergency team. This use of triage differs from that used in wartime as, of course, no patients are left to die after their initial assessment, but the system aims to improve the efficiency of the services offered by an accident and emergency department and ensures that patients are seen according to priority by the correct members of the team. If triage can be shown to work and if health care resources are becoming increasingly scarce, then perhaps it may also be appropriate to adopt a policy of triage for use in treating patients generally.

Triage is used in times of war to treat as many of the casualties as quickly and efficiently as possible in order that the maximum number return to battle in order to achieve the overall objective, that is, to win the war. The fact that some people are denied treatment and left to die is justified by a need to fulfil this overall objective which is considered to be of overriding importance. This is a consequentialist approach to ethics, where it is necessary to consider the possible outcomes of any actions that are taken. Suppose that I believed that participation in the Second World War was justified because, by winning it, the world would be rid of Nazism. It is a necessary part of war that people lose their lives, and although that in itself is not a good thing and to be regretted, I consider it is more beneficial to the world as a whole to remove Hitler from it. So using a policy of triage in wartime does mean that some people are denied treatment, but it may be justified if it means by winning the war something better is achieved.

Justifying the use of triage in other contexts appears to be dependent upon some greater gain for society as a result. It may be argued that triage could be used in peacetime because, by using this system, there would be a more efficient use of health care resources as only those to whom it would be of most benefit would receive treatment. Those treated would then be able to return to their homes, families and jobs, as would those who would get better even without treatment, and only the hopeless cases would die. But would you want human beings to be defined primarily as economic units?

Treating those with the greatest need may be thought of as an efficient use of health care resources, but justification for this method is dependent upon the state of the person's health being the only factor to be taken into consideration, not the person's age, occupation, or position in society. This implies that the seventy-year-old with pneumonia should receive treatment if it will cure him rather than an attempt made to treat a seventeen-year-old victim with severe head injuries following a road accident whose prognosis is very poor. It can be difficult to say exactly whether medical or surgical intervention will save the life of a person and it often is not practical to consider this factor in isolation from other factors such as age or general health which do influence response to treatment.

Justice as fairness

John Rawls, an American philosopher, has put forward in his book *A Theory of Justice* an account of the fairest way that benefits can be distributed within society. Rawls suggests that if people are asked to choose the principles of justice that a society would operate, without knowing what their own position within that society was going to be, they would act in self-interest in order to protect themselves from the worst outcome. This type of selection is made from behind what Rawls calls a 'veil of ignorance', and assumes that people will act rationally. What is suggested would happen in this situation is that people would choose two principles: firstly, that everyone should have equal liberty and secondly, that benefits should be distributed in society so that the worse-off benefit as much as possible and the better-off only benefit if the distribution also benefits the worse-off. This does not mean that Rawls thinks that all people should be treated on an equal basis, but that some inequalities in society will be tolerated if they can be rationally justified.

Suppose that two people require treatment for renal disease: one is a highly skilled surgeon and the other a waiter. There are two treatments available, either renal dialysis, or giving a kidney transplant. Although the first option is an effective treatment, the patient's lifestyle will be severely restricted. The patient will need to be attached to a dialysis machine several times a week and follow strict instructions about what to eat and drink. The patient will probably find it difficult to work either as a surgeon or a waiter if he receives renal dialysis. A kidney transplant is much more successful and guarantees that the patient returns to a normal lifestyle very quickly.

Unfortunately there is only one kidney available for transplant. The options are to select one patient for transplant and treat the other with the poorer treatment, or treat both equally with the poorer treatment. At first sight, the fairest action to take would be to treat both equally with the poorer treatment, but using Rawls's theory it is possible to select the first option and give the surgeon the transplant. This inequality could be tolerated by such a society if in doing so it could be shown that it would benefit the worse-off. If the surgeon is able to return to work after the kidney transplant, then any person in the society requiring surgery (including the worse-off) will benefit. Although the waiter will not be able to

work, it may be argued it would be easier to find someone else to do this
job than to find someone else who is a highly skilled surgeon, and that this
will not affect the worse-off as much as if the surgeon is unable to continue working.

If people had to make this type of selection behind the 'veil of ignorance',
then Rawls's theory suggests that the rational decision would be to select
the surgeon for treatment. In this situation, the worst outcome which these
people need to protect themselves from is either a shortage of waiters or
a shortage of surgeons in the society. As they are unaware of their position
in society and therefore what may happen to them personally, if they act
purely in self-interest it would be more rational to choose a society with
an adequate number of surgeons rather than an adequate number of waiters.

Someone behind the 'veil of ignorance' may argue that he would select
the waiter for the kidney transplant rather than the surgeon, just in case
when the veil is lifted that person discovers that he is to be a waiter. Using
Rawls's theory this would not be a rational choice as by denying the
surgeon the transplant, he is unable to work and again leaves a society
with a shortage of surgeons which would not be in the waiter's interests
should he require further surgery at a later date. The other option would
be to argue for absolute equality of treatment, in this case, to treat both
with renal dialysis, but this would not benefit the worse-off either, as again
it would result in a shortage of skilled surgeons.

However, you could argue that to choose the waiter for the transplant
is still to make a rational choice. As it is likely that there are to be more
waiters than surgeons in society, someone may decide to choose to give the
waiter the transplant, because when the veil is lifted that person knows
that there is far greater likelihood of being a waiter than a surgeon. Such
a decision would be both rational and acting in self-interest.

Another criticism of Rawls's theory discussed by Dworkin concerns the
original position, that is, choosing from behind the veil of ignorance.
Because the two principles seem to be fair, then the original position can
be accepted as an argument to support enforcing these principles, but this
is not so as the following example illustrates.

Suppose that Susan and John share a newspaper round delivering papers
to twelve streets, for which they receive £4 per week. When they receive
their pay on Friday evening, John takes £2.00 and gives £2.00 to Susan.
Susan tells John that she has delivered papers to eight streets whereas he
has only covered four, and so she believes that she is entitled to a greater
share of the money. John disagrees with Susan and thinks that they should
divide the money equally because they took on the paper round as a joint
venture. Susan believes that if she and John had discussed how they were
to share the money before they started the newspaper round, then John
would surely have agreed that the person delivering the most papers would
be entitled to a larger proportion of the money.

If Susan and John had discussed how the money should be divided prior to taking on the paper round, then it is likely that John would have agreed to divide the money according to the number of papers delivered. This would have been a rational decision for him to have made as, if he delivered more newspapers than Susan, he would have felt that he deserved a greater share of the money, and he would therefore have been protecting his own interests. John and Susan (like the people behind Rawls's veil of ignorance) have not made such an agreement. Susan is suggesting that the principle that the money should be divided according to the number of papers delivered is fair. If this principle is fair, then the only reason that John could have for objecting to it is that he will receive less money and so it is contrary to his own self-interest. If it is fair for the money to be divided as Susan suggests, then dividing the money in accordance with that principle will be adequate justification alone. For Susan to support this idea with a hypothetical agreement that she and John might possibly have made is not relevant.

In the same way, if the two principles that Rawls puts forward are fair, then suggesting that people behind the veil of ignorance would also have chosen them is not necessary to support the argument, as the principles should stand up in their own right. Although there are obvious criticisms of Rawls's work, it is worth considering because it does present an alternative to other important types of theories of justice, particularly utilitarian theories.

Treating the greatest number of people

Could or should resources be allocated simply to ensure that as many people as possible are treated? So, for example, if a hospital had £5,000 which could be spent either on giving two patients liver transplants or giving eight people hip replacements, then in order to treat the greatest number, the hip replacements should be carried out at the expense of the liver transplants. This conclusion appears to be harsh on the victims of liver disease who would almost certainly want to know what justification there was for denying them treatment.

There does seem to be some significance attached to numbers; for example, planes that crash or boats that sink resulting in hundreds of deaths are described as tragedies and disasters and usually receive extensive media coverage. On the other hand, we do not use the same type of language to describe the situation if a small plane crashes and only the pilot is killed, nor does the event attract the same amount of media attention. Almost certainly the impact of the death of the pilot is the same on his family and friends as that on the family and friends of a victim of a large plane crash, and it would be odd to be less sympathetic to the family of the lone pilot simply because he was the only person to be killed.

Suppose that I belong to a mountain rescue team that receives two simultaneous calls one evening. One call involves rescuing a party of two walkers, Jim and Jane, and the second is to rescue a single walker, Paul. Apart from knowing how many people are involved, I do not have any further information about them such as their ages or state of health. It is possible to reach with ease both the place where Jim and Jane are, and where Paul is stranded, as neither place is more difficult to get to than the other, but severe weather conditions make it unlikely that the team will be able to reach both places that evening. Any walkers left overnight on the mountain are unlikely to survive the night especially if they are injured. I have to choose whether to try and save both Jim and Jane, or just Paul.

The first matter I may want to decide is if there is any difference between saving one person and saving two. If I decide to go and save Paul, then surely Jim and Jane would not feel that I had harmed them because I had gone to rescue another person. They might well have felt that I had harmed them if I decided the choice was too difficult to make and so went home and left all the walkers stranded. In this situation, all three people can claim that I should treat them as equals, that is, with equal concern and respect. One possible answer to the dilemma is to say that each person counts for one and therefore more than one person counts for more than one. To say otherwise means that extra stranded people count for nothing and have no worth at all. If Paul was stranded and only Jim stranded in another place, although I would still have to make a decision about which of them I would rescue, it would be a very different decision. I could balance the claim that each one had to treatment as an equal, as each would count for one. But Jane also has a claim, and if I decide there is no difference between rescuing two people and rescuing one person, then I am suggesting that Jane does not count for one and as a result her life has no worth at all.

If we accept that each person counts for one, then there is no difficulty justifying hospital expenditure on two liver transplants rather than six hip replacements. Although it seems to make economic sense to treat six people rather than two, if those two people are left with no treatment as a result and face imminent death, then as with Jane stranded on the mountain, it is being suggested that their lives count for nothing at all.

Quality-adjusted life years – QALYs

A great deal of attention is now given to setting standards of care in an attempt to measure the quality of care that patients receive, and at the same time emphasising the need to ensure that the health service is run on efficient lines. Taking this at face value, it seems to be unproblematic. After all, we should want to give patients the treatment that will be of the most benefit to them as well as one that minimises wasting valuable health care resources. It is of course essential to measure efficiency and one system has been devised that measures quality-adjusted life years (QALYs). Use of QALYs has received much attention and provoked debate about whether using this measure can assist in decision-making over the allocation of health care resources.

Using this system, one year of healthy life expectancy counts as one, one year of unhealthy life expectancy counts as less than one, and being dead counts as 0. The exact value is lower the worse the quality of life the person has, but it is possible to have a negative score, that is, less than 0, if the person's quality of life is judged as being worse than dead. Health care is considered to be beneficial if as a result positive QALYs are generated, but health care is considered to be efficient if the cost per QALY is as low as possible. The health economist Alan Williams, who formulated the system, claims that it 'incorporates both life expectancy and quality of life, and . . . reflects the values and ethics of the community served'.

The principle of using QALYs rests on the assumption that if a rational individual was given the choice, that person would prefer to live a shorter life with a minimum amount of suffering and disability as opposed to living for a longer period of time, but with severe disability and suffering. QALYs can then be used in two ways; firstly to decide which amongst a range of treatments is most appropriate for the patient by measuring the net benefit that is expected. So, if there is a choice of two or more possible forms of treatment for a disease, then calculations can be made to find out which one will generate positive QALYs for the patient. Used in this way QALYs can be a useful and ethical way of deciding which treatment may be best for an individual because the focus is on matching the best treatment to the particular patient and does not involve making choices between individuals.

QALYs can also be used in another way when resources are insufficient to meet demand. The same calculations can be made to make decisions about which patients should be treated, and which should be denied treatment. It is this second use of QALYs that is controversial as opponents of the system believe that it allows unfair choices to be made between individuals. Suppose that two people require access to intensive care facilities, but only one bed is available. Calculations can be made to decide how many QALYs will be expected to be generated by treating each patient in the intensive care unit. The patient whose treatment generates the greatest number of positive QALYs would then be treated, although the efficiency of the treatment where the cost per QALY is as low as possible will also be taken into consideration. Using QALYs in this way shifts the focus from deciding what is the best treatment for an individual to deciding which individual is going to benefit most from the treatment available. Although this will undoubtably result in the most efficient use of health care facilities, the system pays no regard to either the claim individuals have to equal treatment or the claim that an individual has to be treated as an equal, and will by definition discriminate against older people.

There is, of course, a need for the health service to be efficient and to ensure that public money is not spent wastefully or inappropriately and it can be argued that it would indeed be unethical for the health service to disregard the importance of this. This is not to say that these factors are the only ones to be taken into consideration when making difficult decisions about the treatment of patients. Although QALYs may be useful in making decisions about which of a choice of treatments will be the most beneficial to an individual, using QALYs to decide which patients to treat and not to treat does not appear to provide the ideal system that its creator suggests, and therefore there is no particular reason to favour its use over any other system of allocating resources.

Self-inflicted illness

A number of patients develop diseases as a direct result of something they have chosen to do to their bodies. The most obvious cases are diseases caused by smoking, alcoholism or drug addiction. However, this group of 'self-inflicted' illnesses could be expanded to include those who have contracted sexually transmitted diseases, individuals who have paid little regard to living a healthy lifestyle with insufficient exercise and an unhealthy diet, and those who engage in dangerous sports. Against a backdrop of diminishing resources, there may appear to be something rather unjust about giving the alcoholic the same chance of a liver transplant as the person who has a non-alcohol-related liver disease, especially if the alcoholic has no intention of trying to stop drinking. But can discrimination against patients with self-inflicted illnesses truly be justified? In some circumstances it may be quite obvious that some action a person has voluntarily taken has resulted in their illness or injury. For example, someone who falls while climbing the north face of the Eiger will sustain injuries directly as a result of taking part in the dangerous sport of mountain climbing. We could then perhaps list the sorts of sports that are considered dangerous and refuse to treat individuals who sustain injuries while engaging in these activities. It would be possible to identify several sports which do have a high incidence of injuries associated with them. But it could be argued that many activities in everyday life also have high incidence of injuries associated with them such as driving a car, climbing on stepladders or crossing a road and these injuries may also be caused by the direct actions of the person who has been injured. The individuals concerned may, for example, have been careless or reckless when driving, failed to secure the stepladders before they stood on them or stepped out in front of traffic on a busy road. Alternatively, the accident may have been caused through no fault of the person who sustained the injuries but completely by accident or perhaps even a combination of the two. In some circumstances it may be in fact impossible to identify the cause of the injuries, particularly if the person is seriously injured and unable to give an explanation or is unconscious. In these situations it would be impractical to try and sort out who sustained injuries as a result of their own actions and deny them treatment, so treatment would have to be given to all. In the same way, those individuals that do engage in dangerous sports will take safety precautions so that they minimise the risk of accidents occurring, and if treatment were to be denied, it would need to be proven that the person had been in some way careless or reckless.

Of course, we could say that people need to cross roads, drive cars and climb ladders as part of their day-to-day activities. We do not need people to climb mountains, visit the South Pole or ski down mountain sides. While this may be true, there is a certain amount of national pride invested in individuals who attain this sort of achievement, and it would necessitate a radical shift in thinking if instead of congratulating individuals on their efforts, it was decided to deny them treatment if they sustained injuries while pursuing these activities. It would also be difficult to say which sort of activities considered unnecessary ran a risk of causing injury to the participants, as it is likely that more people will be injured as a result of playing soccer or rugby than by engaging in what are thought to be more dangerous sports. Mountain climbers and the like may consider it unjust that players of an equally unnecessary sport should have their injuries treated simply because it is not considered to be as dangerous as mountain climbing!

The same difficulties are encountered when trying to sort out the causes of other diseases which are associated with smoking, alcohol consumption or an unhealthy lifestyle. Although it can be shown that there are direct links between these diseases and causative factors, we cannot say that every case of lung cancer is caused by the person smoking cigarettes because such a statement is simply false. This is particularly true of factors associated with diet. Advice that was given to previous generations about which foods were healthy to eat, such as dairy products, and which to avoid, like pasta, potatoes and bread, is completely contrary to what we consider to be good dietary advice in the 1990s.

There is a much larger question behind this issue which is – are we entitled to restrict people's freedom to live the sort of lifestyle they want to, particularly if they are not harming others as a result? It is difficult to give clear reasons why we should restrict individuals' lifestyles, particularly as there would be few of us whose lifestyle would hold up to scrutiny in fine detail. It is even more difficult to imagine how such restrictions would be controlled. Would people be rationed as to how much alcohol, animal fat, or whatever current science showed to be dangerous things, to consume? Would health professionals have to report the illnesses and injuries people had to some higher authority who would decide if they might be treated or not? A system that decided which people should be denied treatment as a result of their own actions would have vast implications upon society and could be as costly to administer as treating the people in the first case.

The case studies

In light of this discussion, let us look back at the case studies. In the case of Ben, the physically and mentally disabled child, he needs intensive care facilities to treat a chest infection. The consultant in charge of the unit objects to Ben's admission as he feels that Ben has a poor quality of life and that there are more deserving cases. By giving these two reasons, Dr Nelson is not just refusing to treat Ben because he feels that Ben is a hopeless case, but he thinks that others deserve to have the bed rather than Ben. If Dr Nelson wanted to deny Ben treatment simply because he felt that it was not worth it, then the number of beds available on the intensive care unit would be of no relevance. Dr Nelson might well argue that if resources were not a problem, then he would not feel that he had to discriminate against someone like Ben. He is forced to make these difficult decisions only because of limited resources. If this is true, then a decision about who should have the bed must be made by looking at other relevant issues.

As described above, there are several different ways of deciding who should be given the bed and not just which person is thought to be in greatest need. It would be possible to argue that Ben should be given the bed because he was there first. Dr Nelson believes that there will be others who will require the bed the following day, but there does not appear to be any other patient needing the bed at the present time. Mr and Mrs Yates may feel that it would be unjust to deny Ben treatment because someone else may need the bed at a later date. Ben's parents could, on his behalf, claim that Ben has a right to be treated as an equal, and to deny him the bed and give it to someone else is not respecting that claim.

What seems to be crucial is that Ben is seen to have a poor quality of life, and Dr Nelson thinks that even if he gives Ben the bed, it will make no appreciable difference to his life in general. While this may be true from Dr Nelson's perspective, it is most unlikely that Mr and Mrs Yates will agree with him. An important point is who should ultimately be given the final decision in this case – should it be Dr Nelson, or should the parents be able to decide what form of treatment their child should have? Although parents should be, and are usually, involved in the decision-making process, the courts have tended to defer to medical opinion and in effect often override the wishes of the parents.

If Dr Nelson does refuse to treat Ben because of his poor quality of life, he will need to say exactly why he thinks that saving Ben is a waste of time. This will have implications for the decisions he may make about other disabled people in the future. Dr Nelson could justify this by saying that although he would not discriminate against disabled people in normal circumstances, the circumstances he finds himself in are far from normal and he has to find a solution to allocating life-saving resources when they are scarce. However, selecting disabled people as a group to discriminate against could be seen as arbitrary, and Dr Nelson would need not only to be able to demonstrate why this is the correct group to select, but also to explain how he will differentiate between disabled and non-disabled people. Would he, for example, consider someone severely physically and mentally disabled like Ben in the same category as someone physically disabled due to rheumatoid arthritis whose quality of life is physically also poor, but who remains mentally very alert?

In our other case study, a young man with AIDS has requested admission to a hospice. Sister Dunne wants to deny Peter access to the hospice, as she argues that to admit him would damage relations between the general public and the hospice. This may well be true, as there appears to be a great deal of misunderstanding and ignorance about AIDS in society, but the hospice management committee will need to assess how real this threat is. As the hospice depends upon charity and voluntary workers, it could be argued that it would be pointless to admit patients with AIDS if, as a result, funding was severely restricted.

As in the previous case, Peter can claim to have a right to equal treatment and also claim a right to be treated as an equal, and by denying him treatment neither claim is being recognised. Peter may therefore feel that denying him access to what is considered the best treatment available because of the nature of his illness is unjust. The hospice management committee would need therefore to demonstrate that an institution dependent upon charity was justified in acting in this way if its existence was threatened as a result. If Dr Wall insists on admitting Peter and the hospice experiences financial difficulties, it may be argued that he is failing to respect the claim that others in the future may lose out on equal treatment if they cannot be given access to the facilities of the hospice.

Although the issue of self-inflicted illness is not voiced, because of the sort of misunderstandings that exist in society about this disease, it may be relevant to consider whether this is the real reason why admitting individuals with AIDS would be frowned upon, especially in a hospice with religious links. While a religious group may feel that they can make general statements about moral issues, it should be accepted that these only hold for the adherents to that particular group. In this case the hospice committee may feel that it is entitled to admit only those patients whom it chooses to care for, but this would also show discrimination against sections of the community that fund-raisers might find unacceptable and might still lead to financial difficulties.

Health care resources and law

If considerations of justice are at the heart of the debate on allocation of health care resources, you might expect the law to play a major role in that debate. You would be wrong. The courts are unwilling to intervene in disputes on allocation of resources or prioritisation of treatments. The law's role is generally limited to checking manifest injustice. However, as in so many areas of health care law, change is coming and, as we shall see, English judges are beginning at least to recognise the crucial importance of resource questions.

For the lawyer the core of the resource issue is simply this. Is there a right to health care and, if so, who is subject to a duty to provide that care and how is that duty enforced? A moral right to health care seems undebatable. The ethical imperative to treat the sick has been taken for granted in the first sections of this chapter. Article 25 of the United Nations Declaration of Human Rights asserts a right to adequate medical care. What substance does English law give to that 'right'?

The National Health Service Act 1977 imposes on the Secretary of State for Health a duty to continue the promotion of 'a comprehensive health service' and to provide, to such extent as he considers necessary to meet all reasonable requirements, services including medical, nursing and dental services, and hospital accommodation. So if the Minister falls short in his duties relating to the macro-allocation of resources, and fails to provide enough cash for a particular type of treatment, will the courts intervene? In *R v. Secretary of State for Social Services ex p. Hincks* (1979) an all-too-common scenario occurred. Mr Hincks and three other patients needed orthopaedic surgery. They had been waiting for ages and the longer they waited the more the prospects for a successful outcome diminished. They went to court asking for compensation for pain and suffering and an order that the Minister provide their health authority with the money to enable surgery to take place more or less straight away. Both claims failed.

The Court of Appeal gave the following rulings. Firstly, the duty to provide services was a duty owed to all of us collectively, not as individual patients. An individual injured through lack of care could not demand damages and harsh though this sounds it may be sensible. Money paid out of the NHS budget to meet A's claim for damages could mean no money to pay for treatment of B and C. What will be the effect of current government plans to 'fine' NHS trusts who fail to meet treatment targets? Secondly, the Minister's duty to provide services was limited by the budget for total health care he received from the Treasury. His decisions as to how to share out that budget could only be reviewed by the courts if shown to be improperly motivated or wholly outrageous or unreasonable. So if a Liberal Democrat Minister declared that only Liberal Democrats should receive NHS care, or if he or she opined that Southerners were too rich for free care, so that 90 per cent of the NHS budget would be allocated to north of Birmingham, in those exceptional cases, the courts could be invoked to outlaw manifest injustice.

Would an attempt to enforce a claim to health care be more successful if aimed at a local health authority (or whatever body constitutes the local 'purchaser' charged with arranging health care in their area)? Precedent suggests not. In two cases in Birmingham (*R* v. *Central Birmingham HA ex p. Walker and ex p. Collier*), parents of infants with congenital heart defects went to court seeking orders that their babies be given priority for surgery. Both infants were undoubtedly very ill and would be listed for surgery, only to be 'bumped down' the queue because an even more urgent 'emergency' case was admitted. The problem was that Birmingham lacked enough trained paediatric nurses to treat all the babies in clinical need of treatment. The Court of Appeal refused to intervene. Judges could not determine clinical priorities. There was no evidence that the treatment decisions made in the light of shortage of resources were manifestly unreasonable. One of the judges expressed fears that if patients whose treatment was denied or delayed regularly resorted to the courts, litigation costs would eat into the health authority budget, aggravating those shortages.

In both the above sets of cases, the courts refused to intervene to upset judgments made on clinical bases. What if a judgment to refuse treatment is based on non-clinical criteria? Perhaps renal dialysis is offered only to patients under seventy, or smokers are denied bypass surgery. Will judges feel more confident to adjudicate on the propriety or otherwise of that sort of social criteria? In *R* v. *St. Mary's Hospital Ethical Advisory Committee ex p. Harriott*, Mrs Harriott had been rejected for treatment in the hospital's *in vitro* fertilisation programme. Enquiries had revealed that she had a conviction for prostitution-related offences and had been found unsuitable as a potential adoptive or foster parent by Manchester City Council. She sought to challenge the hospital's decision. The judge said that in the context of the treatment she wanted, her suitability as a parent was a factor which the clinician deciding whether to treat her could lawfully consider. But he stressed that firstly, anybody making decisions about whom to treat must act on fair and relevant criteria and secondly, unjustifiable discrimination was unlawful. Refusal of treatment based on sex, race or religion would clearly be struck down by the courts. Other obviously irrelevant criteria for choice would also be unlawful. For example, if Mrs Harriott needed treatment for cervical cancer, to refuse her care on the basis of her past would almost certainly be unlawful.

Do not expect the courts to be radical in their approach to resource decisions. Powerful evidence of something approaching bad faith may be necessary before the law steps in to halt injustice. That the courts are only too aware of the problems of resources is illustrated by this quotation from a judgment of Lord Donaldson refusing parents an order requiring doctors to give their dying babies treatment which the doctors believed to be futile. He said courts must

> take account of the sad fact of life that health authorities on occasions find that they may have too few resources, either human or material or both, to treat all the patients they would like to treat in the way in which they would like to treat them. (*Re J* (1992) p. 517)

7

Responsibilities and accountability

As a registered, nurse, midwife or health visitor, you are personally accountable for your practice. (Introduction to Code of Professional Conduct)

Personally accountable

Each and every one of us will be held to account by the law if, by our
carelessness, we injure a person whom we have a duty to protect from
harm. So if you drive your car carelessly and knock down a pedestrian on
a pelican crossing when the lights are on red, the law will order you to
compensate that pedestrian for his injuries. If as a nurse you carelessly fail
to put up the cotsides of the bed of a demented and restless patient, you
will be liable if he falls out of bed and breaks a hip. The law demands
nurses attain and maintain professional standards of practice. What constitutes professional standards is left largely to the profession itself to
determine. The UKCC regulates nursing practice in this country, and describes the *Code of Professional Conduct* as its definitive statement on
professional conduct. It sets the standard against which allegations of
misconduct will be measured. There is also a moral dimension to accountability for practice, particularly so when conflicts occur, for example,
between different health professionals, between senior and junior staff, or
when there is an enlargement in the scope of a nurse's personal professional practice. The following case studies illustrate this moral dimension
of accountability.

The doubting junior nurse

Sue Robinson, an enrolled nurse, is often in charge of a medical ward on
night duty. Peter Smith is the night charge nurse responsible for the ward
that Sue works on and the coronary care unit. One night Peter visits the
ward when Sue is on duty, and informs her that the coronary care unit has
run out of Diamorphine injections, and that it will be necessary to take an
ampoule from her ward stock to the coronary care unit.

Diamorphine is both a very strong analgesic and a controlled drug. It is a legal requirement that the number of stock ampoules be recorded in a special register. Each administration of the drug must be to a named patient who is recorded in the register and signed by the nurse who administers the drug and by a second nurse who witnesses it being given. On this occasion, Sue fills out the register with the name of the patient on the coronary care unit that Peter informs her requires the Diamorphine. Peter signs as the nurse who administers the drug and tells Sue to sign the register to show that she has witnessed it being given.

Sue feels unhappy about doing this, as she is aware that she will not witness the drug being given. She is alone on the ward and cannot leave without arranging for a nurse from another ward to come and cover for her. This would take time and prolong the period that the patient is in pain. Sue also feels unsure about challenging Peter's authority on this matter as he has told her to sign the register. To refuse will imply that she does not trust him to administer the drug to the patient. As Peter is in a far more senior position than Sue he may be affronted by such a challenge and this could damage working relations with him in future.

Pressures at home and work

Sister Clark, aged fifty-three, has worked for over thirty years in a district hospital and is respected amongst staff and patients. For the last twelve years she has been in charge of ward five and has made it known that she intends to continue working on the ward until she retires at fifty-five. She has always taken her role as ward sister seriously and has devised a comprehensive teaching programme for students allocated to her ward. She is renowned for her efficiency in ward management, staff allocation and stock control.

Four months ago Sister Clark's husband suffered a stroke and was admitted to hospital. Eventually Mr Clark was discharged but is seriously disabled by the stroke and needs assistance with all basic human needs. Although she has been given help from social services, Sister Clark has found it increasingly difficult to cope with the demands of a full-time job and a heavily dependent husband. She is frequently late for duty and has found it necessary to take extra time off to care for her husband.

Mrs Pearson, the surgical unit manager, is aware of the problems that are beginning to develop on the ward. June Young, the junior sister, has taken over responsibility for teaching the students, the off-duty rota and stock ordering, but has made it known to Mrs Pearson that she considers it unfair that Sister Clark is still recognised and paid as the senior sister. Mrs Pearson is also concerned that the situation on the ward is preventing adequate nursing care being given to the patients at all times. Mrs Pearson knows that if Sister Clark stops working before she is fifty-five, she will lose superannuation benefits.

Mrs Pearson is aware that despite everything Sister Clark is still a popular figure, and many feel sympathy with the situation that she is now in. Mrs Pearson has recently discussed Sister Clark's domestic difficulties with her and made some alternative suggestions such as reducing her hours at work, or allowing June Young to take over as 'acting senior sister'. Sister Clark rejected these suggestions saying that she needed to work full-time and that she intended to remain in charge until retirement.

Mrs Pearson is faced with either accepting Sister Clark's position until her retirement – thereby compromising patient care and possibly causing difficulties amongst the other ward staff – or disregarding her long record of good service, and instigating disciplinary action against her for not fulfilling her role as senior sister. This may result in Sister Clark being dismissed, causing her financial difficulties and risking public outrage.

Ethical considerations: responsibility

In Chapter Five, the duty of confidentiality was described, using H. L. A. Hart's definition of 'role responsibility'. For a nurse, role responsibility means she is responsible for fulfilling whatever duties are recognised as part of her role as a nurse. A duty to respect confidences is only one of the many professional responsibilities that a nurse may be said to have which may vary according to the working environment. The role of a nurse working on a hospital ward, for example, will include responsibilities such as administering medication and treatment, maintaining records and perhaps teaching students, whereas the role of a practice nurse working in a health centre may have quite different responsibilities such as advising on health promotion or giving vaccinations. Whatever the circumstances, a nurse will have a recognised role and corresponding responsibilities attached to it.

Role responsibility can be thought of as either legal or moral. It could be said, for example, that a nurse has a contractual responsibility to be on duty according to the duty rota unless she has reasonable excuse, and when her span of duty is finished she is entitled to go off duty. But suppose that during the course of the day Helen, a registered nurse on a female surgical ward, has been caring for Christine, a patient scheduled for surgery that afternoon. Christine is extremely apprehensive about being anaesthetised. In order to reassure Christine, Helen has said that she will personally take Christine to theatre and stay until she has had the anaesthetic administered. If Helen's shift finishes before Christine is called to theatre, Helen may feel she has a responsibility to fulfil her promise to Christine, but this is not a legal responsibility. Having finished her allotted span of duty Helen has satisfied her contractual requirements. However, it could be argued that she has a moral responsibility to keep the promise and so she may decide to stay on duty to do so. We can describe Helen as a responsible nurse, a person who takes her duties seriously, thinks about them and makes serious efforts to fulfil them.

Nurses, then, are responsible for their actions according to the role that they play within society, but there are some exceptions to this, for example, if a nurse is mentally ill, or is coerced by others into acting in a way that she would not usually agree with.

Accountability

Being called to account simply means being asked to give reasons for your actions. As part of everyday life people are often called to account for their actions in a legal, moral or completely neutral capacity. A police officer may ask you to account for having parked your car on a double yellow line; your friend, having found out that you have lied to her may call you to account for it; or your partner may ask you to account for having hung a picture on one wall rather than the other. In each situation it is possible to give reasons for your actions which may range from very good reasons to none at all.

If someone is called to account in a legal or moral capacity, then it is because they have carried out some action that is not allowed, is unacceptable or is unusual, and they may incur penalties as a result of their actions. The purpose of calling to account in this way is to establish whether a person has good enough reasons for acting in the way they did. The person who parked their car on the double yellow line may be a doctor who has been called urgently to the house of a critically ill patient, or could just have stopped outside a shop to buy groceries. Although the action is illegal, the police officer may decide to ignore the doctor's car, but give a parking ticket in the latter instance. In a similar way, you may have very good reasons or poor reasons for lying to your friend. If your friend accepts your reasons, then no penalties are incurred; if, however, she does not, then you may risk losing her friendship or becoming known as an untrustworthy person.

Nurses are responsible for carrying out the duties considered to be part of their professional role. As a result they are accountable for their actions as professionals which the UKCC considers then to be at all times 'whether engaged in current practice or not and whether on or off duty'.

A nurse may be held to account legally and/or morally for whatever actions she is responsible for. So a nurse, having decided upon a course of action, should be able to give reasons for choosing to act in that way rather than selecting any other course of action.

We distinguished Helen's moral responsibilities from her contractual responsibilities. Having defined her responsibilities we can now consider how Helen can be held accountable. If Helen decides to stay on duty and take Christine to theatre and is called to account, she could cite a belief in a moral responsibility to the patient. Alternatively, if she decides to go off duty on time and breaks her promise to Christine she may or may not be able to give very good reasons for doing so.

Legally, even if she broke her promise, Helen fulfilled her contractual requirements. The situation is more complex if she is to account morally for her actions. Although it is unlikely that Helen would receive any formal sort of disciplinary action for breaking her promise, she could incur other sanctions such as being considered unreliable or not taking her responsibilities seriously.

Historically, nurses have not been encouraged to make and act upon their own clinical or moral judgments and have, perhaps, been actively discouraged from doing so. The nurse's role in caring for patients was to carry out the orders of the doctors who made the decisions about patient care. Within this setting, nurses were accountable to the person making those decisions, namely the doctor or perhaps the employing institution. This sort of perception of the nurse's role is clearly documented in international codes of practice prior to the early 1970s. The emphasis then changed and nurses, instead of having an obligation to carry out a doctor's orders, became accountable to those individuals requiring nursing care, that is, the clients and patients. Nurses in this country are expected to carry this responsibility one step further and accept a role of patient advocate.

A nurse is therefore responsible for the care she gives to patients and is accountable to them for her actions according to the standard of practice expected by the UKCC. It is, however, important to note that it is regard for the interests of clients and patients that should ultimately govern a nurse's professional practice and not regard for the rules of the UKCC. It is necessary to have the emphasis this way round to guard against what may be thought of as defensive practice.

Defensive practice

Defensive practice means allowing a fear of criticism, media exposure or, in extreme cases, litigation, to dictate what form of treatment a patient may receive regardless of whether it is the most appropriate form of treatment for that particular individual. This may take the form of any sort of ritualised investigations or treatment being given to a patient which will be of little benefit and costly to society in general. The increase in the Caesarean section rate in the United States has caused concern and may possibly be explained as an example of defensive practice.

It has been suggested that the rise in Caesarean sections is due to the fact that doctors fear being sued by their patients if a baby suffers from mental or physical damage that could be linked to their mode of delivery. It is argued that birth trauma is less likely to occur if a Caesarean section is performed rather than, for example, a forceps delivery. For this reason some doctors are more inclined to perform a Caesarean section. There is of course nothing morally dubious about a practitioner making a clinical judgment on the evidence that is before her or him, as long as the judgments are made solely in the interests of the patient. Difficulties arise when the practitioner makes a clinical judgment that places her or his own interests above those of the patient.

There are also instances in clinical practice where nurses may exhibit defensive practice. Health care litigation is on the increase and many health professionals now fear that they are ever more likely to be sued if they make a mistake. Defensive practice has become an issue amidst these fears. Nurses are frequently urged to record problems or adverse events in a patient's nursing notes to 'cover themselves'. For example, a nurse in charge of a ward who believes that there are insufficient staff to care for the number of patients may report this to the line manager. If no further staff are available, the nurse may document that he has requested more staff in the event that care is compromised and litigation ensues. It is undoubtedly important that such information is documented, but if the sole reason for doing so is to protect the nurse's interests, it may be argued that this is defensive practice.

Successful medical suits and large compensation awards receive great media and public attention and it is true that patients are more willing to sue today than they were twenty years ago. Despite this, fears of a 'malpractice crisis' and subsequent defensive practice are not justified. Legal suits are extremely costly and a patient who loses faces paying the legal costs of the other party. Few people are wealthy enough to fund a medical law suit and legal aid is available only to the small number of people who fall below the extremely low financial threshold. Furthermore, the granting of such financial aid often depends on the likelihood of success. As you will see from this chapter and Chapter Four, the plaintiff's chances of success in court are relatively small and it can take years before a court comes to a decision. When faced with all this, a patient must assess whether the compensation he may or may not win is worth the trauma and expense. Minor injuries receive small compensation – most patients will not bother or will not be able to afford to sue.

This does not answer the nurse's moral problem. Where patient care may still be compromised in practice, the nurse may be unable to do anything more than inform the line manager. The line manager's role is to ensure adequate staffing levels for clinical areas; if she is also a nurse then she would be held personally accountable for failing to respond to this request. All nurses, midwives and health visitors are bound by the *Code of Professional Conduct*, irrespective of their seniority.

Why act morally?

Dilemmas may occur in clinical practice when the nurse knows what the morally correct course of action should be, but fear of recrimination prevents her from following her instincts. Suppose Kate, a registered nurse, makes an error when administering drugs to a patient, and gives two ferrous sulphate tablets instead of one. Although there is a possiblity that the patient may suffer ill effects as a result, Kate knows that this is unlikely. However, she is aware that if she confesses to having made this error, she will be severely reprimanded and humiliated. Kate may feel that although the patient may suffer, she knows that she is almost certainly going to suffer more as a consequence of admitting to the error, so why should she own up? The *Code of Professional Conduct* clearly states that nurses should ensure that no action or omission on their part is detrimental to the condition of patients. But to use this clause of the Code as a reason for admitting responsibility suggests defensive practice. It is necessary therefore to find a more substantial reason to answer the question.

Within moral philosophy there are many different and diverse theories about morality and ideas as to how these theories may be applied to everyday life. Most ethical theories, however, agree that moral principles are universal. This does not mean that particular moral principles can be applied in every case, as circumstances may cause them to change. Take for example the moral principle, 'lying is wrong'. It would be difficult to say that this principle can be universally applied in every case as there may be circumstances when lying is not considered wrong. We would not, for example, morally condemn Germans who lied to the Nazis about the Jews they hid in their homes simply because they were being dishonest. To say that 'lying is wrong' is a universal moral principle means that lying can never be justified according to an individual's personal preferences or prejudices.

If Kate says nothing and the patient does not suffer as a result of the error, she may be justified in keeping quiet. Although she is acting in self-interest she is not necessarily compromising the patient's interests. Take another example. Suppose your elderly bedridden aunt has given you a china vase which has great sentimental value for her. Unfortunately you break it. You know that she would be upset if she knew the vase was broken and would reprimand you for being careless. As your aunt is housebound and will not find out, you decide not to tell her. You could be said to be acting according to your own interests, but your behaviour would not necessarily be described as immoral simply because you have not admitted breaking the vase when your aunt will not suffer as a result (but you would be reprimanded if you told her). In the same way, if the patient has not suffered, it may be argued that there seems little to gain by Kate owning up to her error. It is far more likely that a nurse in Kate's position would be shocked by her mistake and resolve to be more careful in future, thereby punishing herself.

If, however, the patient's condition deteriorates as a result of Kate's error, but she decides not to admit to it because she is afraid of being disciplined, then Kate will have greater difficulty justifying her position. It may be argued that she is acting according to her own interests or preferences and consequently is choosing to disregard those of the patient. It is not possible to believe that moral principles are universal whilst simultaneously defending an action according to whatever moral principle an individual prefers at any given time. If Kate puts her own interests over those of the patient then clearly she thinks that moral principles are not universal and that she may act according to what benefits her in every instance.

By definition it seems unlikely that a nurse could be satisfied with this outcome as she must surely be concerned about the interests of other people to enter the profession in the first place. In this instance, Kate should admit to making an error because she is unable to defend self-interest as an overriding moral principle. This is also the course of action suggested by the *Code of Professional Conduct*.

Professional competence

It may seem obvious that nurses should be competent to practise, and an important part of this is keeping up to date with current practice in nursing. Although many nurses keep up to date by reading journals and attending study days and conferences, it is possible for a nurse, once qualified, to avoid any form of continuing education for the rest of his or her career. The *Code of Professional Conduct* also states that a nursing professional should 'maintain and improve . . . professional knowledge and competence'. At present, only midwives have a statutory requirement to attend a five-day refresher course, five approved study days every five years or another approved course to maintain their practising status.

In 1990, the UKCC developed the Post-registration Education and Practice Project (PREPP), which outlined proposals for support for newly qualified nurses, the development of nurse practitioners and consultants, a return-to-practice programme for nurses who have had a break of five years or more from practice and proposals for continuing education. PREPP proposes that nurses should be obliged to have five days study leave every three years and also that nurses should demonstrate that they have maintained and developed their professional knowledge and competence. The precise nature of these proposals has not yet been specified and is currently under discussion.

It may be thought that these proposals do not go far enough to ensure that nurses are competent in their clinical practice, but considering that there is no statutory obligation for nurses to up date themselves at present, these proposals will surely help to improve the situation. Of course it may be argued that nurses should have some sort of moral obligation to be responsible for their own standards of practice in order to maintain high standards in the clinical area. While this may be true, if the nursing profession's commitment to professional competence is to be taken seriously, then a more structured form of continuing education is also needed.

Keeping abreast of current practice and developments is equally important in legal terms. The common law requires that a nurse conform to 'accepted practice'. This concept is examined in detail later on, but a minimum requirement is that a nurse should read material which is readily available to all nurses – failure to read one specific article or obscure publication will not be legally condemned. Neither can a nurse be sanctioned retrospectively if the current practice of the time proves later to be defective.

Working within the health care team – patient advocacy

Nurses work in multi-disciplinary teams. They plan and implement care on their own initiative as well as participating in the care provided by others in the health care team such as doctors, physiotherapists, and other therapists. Ideally all members of the health care team should collaborate to ensure that patients receive the best treatment possible in the most practical and efficient manner, so that doctors make decisions about medical treatment and nurses make decisions about nursing care with dialogue between the two professions. However, there are instances when the situation is less than ideal, and this is most likely to occur if individual members of the team refuse to respect or acknowledge the skills and opinions of other members.

As a member of a team a nurse's accountability can be seen in two ways. First, in the ideal situation where he is able to make decisions and influence change, the nurse will be able to justify the actions that he has taken in a professional capacity. Unfortunately, some nurses work in conditions falling far short of that ideal and in these situations their accountability can be viewed differently. A consultant may see herself as ultimately in charge of the patients under her care and believe that she should make or approve all decisions that are made regarding the patient. A nurse working on the ward with such a consultant may feel that he has no influence over the treatment the patient receives. Whilst in the worst possible circumstances this may be true, working within a team does not absolve a nurse of his individual responsibility and accountability for practice.

Suppose a nurse working in this situation discovers that a patient has been prescribed twice the normal dose of a drug. Although he is dubious he gives it anyway, claiming that his only responsibility is to administer drugs as prescribed by the doctor. If the dose is incorrect, this nurse considers that it is the doctor's fault and not his. This stance conflicts with the idea of a nurse as an autonomous practitioner and patient advocate. The UKCC encourages nurses to act as advocates for patients and defines advocacy as being 'concerned with promoting the well-being and interests of patients and clients'. It cannot be in a patient's interests for a nurse to suspect that he is giving an incorrect dose of a drug. The correct course of action for him to take would be to query the dosage with the prescribing doctor. The nurse remains morally and legally accountable for his own actions and if he fails to clarify the situation, then it must be assumed that either he has good reasons for giving the drug or has chosen to disregard the fact that he is accountable. He will have difficulty justifying either option.

In acting as advocate for his patient, and on questioning the doctor, the nurse may find that there is a good reason for the prescription. If the nurse is satisfied with the explanation he may decide to administer the drug as prescribed. However, it may be that the doctor has made an error in writing the prescription and so by acting as advocate the nurse has prevented unnecessary suffering for the patient. Alternatively, the doctor may fail to give the nurse a satisfactory reason but tell him to give the dose anyway. If so, the nurse may give the drug, but record the events in the nursing records indicating that although he challenged the doctor, he was instructed to give the drug as prescribed. This may fulfil his legal obligations, but is it morally questionable?

It would not make sense for a nurse acting as patient advocate to disregard his own misgivings and administer the drug, because even though the doctor has instructed him to proceed he still remains accountable for his actions. If he takes his role seriously, then unless he is given good reasons for giving the drug he cannot be said to be safeguarding the well-being of this patient. It may be argued that his position is no different from that of the nurse who thinks that it is not his responsibility and gives the drug without question.

Although it is essential that accurate nursing records are kept on all aspects of patient care, this does not remove the moral responsibility for safeguarding a patient's well-being. It is in every nurse's interest to ensure that he keeps accurate records; should the need arise for him to account in a legal framework then he will be able to do so. However, further analysis is necessary if a nurse is to satisfy the moral dimension of accountability and responsibility.

The ethical dilemmas for Sue Robinson and Mrs Pearson

Peter Smith in the case study is a charge nurse and therefore is senior to Sue Robinson. Traditionally hospitals have been run on hierarchical lines and junior members of staff have been discouraged from questioning the actions or orders of senior staff. Times have changed and in current nursing practice there seems little justification for this. If a nurse is accountable for her practice as an individual then there may be occasions when it is necessary for her to question those in positions of seniority about their actions if there is any doubt. Sue, therefore, should not sign the register saying that she has witnessed the Diamorphine being given simply because Peter has told her to do so.

Sue has two options. She can disregard the rules governing the use of controlled drugs, as Peter has suggested, sign the register and therefore avoid confronting him. Alternatively, she may refuse to comply with Peter's suggestion and arrange for another nurse to be present on the ward in her absence. Each outcome is equally undesirable. By following the first option Sue is acting illegally, and by following the second, she will leave the patient in pain for a longer period of time.

If Sue follows the first course of action in order to avoid damaging her working relationship with Peter, it may be argued that she is acting according to her personal preferences rather than a wider moral principle. This is a difficult position for a nurse to justify. Sue could argue that she acted in this way because she does not want the patient to suffer unnecessary pain and is therefore acting in the patient's interests. To defend this position Sue will need to demonstrate that acting in the patient's interests in this way overrides the legal rules concerning controlled drugs, which will be difficult. Although the patient will be left in pain for longer, it seems that Sue really has little alternative than to administer the medication following the correct procedure. This solution is far from ideal but appears to be the best option to take. As is often the case, when a nurse like Sue is faced with a moral dilemma, there may not be one completely satisfactory solution. One way of solving these sorts of problems is to weigh up the options and decide which one is closest to the ideal.

Mrs Pearson in the second case study has a conflict between sympathy for her colleague Sister Clark, and her professional responsibility as a manager. She sympathises with Sister Clark and does not want to make matters any worse for her. But, as alternative solutions have been rejected, Mrs Pearson is faced with the decision either to take disciplinary action against Sister Clark, in view of her recent conduct, or to ignore the situation on the ward.

Mrs Pearson could first analyse why she is reluctant to take disciplinary action against Sister Clark. If she is concerned that she will be criticised by those who sympathise with Sister Clark it may be argued that Mrs

Pearson is acting according to her own preferences in order to protect her own interests. The difficulty in justifying such preferences has been a recurring theme in this chapter. If, however, Mrs Pearson wants to avoid causing more problems for Sister Clark it may be argued that she is acting to protect Sister Clark's interests and she may find this easier to defend. This is, of course, only half the story. Mrs Pearson may have discovered why she is reluctant to take disciplinary action against Sister Clark but she still does not know if she can justify her decision.

Mrs Pearson is concerned that the situation on the ward is preventing adequate nursing care being given to the patients at all times. As the surgical unit nurse manager, Mrs Pearson may see an area of conflict between the needs of the patients and the needs of the staff, and she must consider her role in protecting the interests of the patients. Mrs Pearson is both a manager and a nurse, and thus bound by the UKCC's *Code of Professional Conduct*. In its document *Exercising Accountability*, the UKCC states that 'the individual nurse, midwife or health visitor should recognise that the interests of public and patient must predominate over those of practitioner and profession'. In order to act according to the *Code of Professional Conduct*, Mrs Pearson must view the patient's interests as the most important factor in this case. If Mrs Pearson decides to ignore the situation on the ward to protect Sister Clark's interests, thereby compromising patients' well-being, she will need to justify not only placing Sister Clark's interests above those of the patients but her disregard of the *Code of Professional Conduct*.

Responsibility and accountability in law

Any person who professes to have a special skill or training upon which others rely will be in a position of responsibility and may therefore be held legally accountable for their actions.

The UKCC is statutorily obliged to regulate the conduct and practices of nursing professionals and through its *Code of Professional Conduct* sets standards for nurses that are often higher and more demanding than existing legal standards.

Accountability of nursing professionals may be achieved in a number of ways such as the following:

1. An aggrieved patient or colleague may complain to the UKCC resulting in a hearing before the Professional Conduct Committee.
2. A patient may complain formally using the Hospital Complaints Procedure to ask the NHS Commissioner for a review.
3. A complaint made to the nurse's employer may result in disciplinary procedures and a tribunal hearing.

4.   The patient may sue the nurse for any breach of her many legal duties
     and responsibilities.

The relationship between moral accountability and the UKCC code of
ethics has already been discussed. The main focus for the remaining part
of this chapter is on the legal responsibility and accountability of the
nurse. In Chapter Three you were introduced to a number of areas of law
which are relevant to nursing practice. By far the most important area of
law in terms of accountability is the civil law of tort. The law of tort is
designed to provide complainants with compensation for the harm they
have suffered by either negligence or some other wrongdoing. Where an
action in tort is brought, the nurse is being asked to account to the patient
and the court for her actions.

The most common actions in health care litigation are negligence claims
and claims for trespass to the person. Although compensation is often
stated to be the primary objective of the law of tort, many patients com-
mence law suits in order to discover what actually happened and to enforce accountability of the responsible professionals. The tort of battery
was discussed in Chapter Four and is crucial to questions of consent, but
legal accountability will often be sought in actions for negligence.

Negligence is a failure on the part of one person to take reasonable care
which causes foreseeable damage to another. In law it means more than
carelessness – not every act of carelessness which causes harm will give rise
to a successful claim in negligence. The plaintiff-patient must prove three
main elements before a nurse will be judged to have been negligent. First,
he must prove that the defendant nurse and/or health authority owed him
a duty of care. Second, he must prove that the defendant breached that
duty (i.e. that she was in fact negligent). Finally, it must be proven that the
injuries of which he complains were actually caused by the nurse's negligence – this is known as causation, and is often the greatest difficulty
confronted in medical negligence claims.

1. The legal duty of care

Put very simply, a duty of care in law generally arises when a person can
reasonably foresee that careless conduct is likely to cause physical injury
or damage to another person or to property. Whether or not the injury is
foreseeable is decided by the courts and depends on the relationship between the parties. Foreseeability of injury clearly exists within the nurse-
patient relationship and it is well established that all health practitioners
owe their patients a duty of care.

Conduct can include both acts and omissions but in general there is no
duty to intervene to help or treat another person unless there is some pre-
existing relationship, i.e. he is a patient in your ward or part of your

practice. In other words there is no duty to be a Good Samaritan. A nurse is under no legal obligation to go to the aid of an accident victim if she happens to be walking by on her day off. If, however, she does offer help she creates a duty relationship and may be held liable if she negligently causes more damage.

Once someone is accepted as a patient then failing to treat him is as much legally actionable as any careless act. If a health visitor fails to visit a sick infant on her list she is as much liable for omitting to provide care as if she negligently caused harm by some foolish act. In *Barnett* v. *Chelsea and Kensington HMC* (1969) Mr Barnett was admitted to casualty after being violently sick. The casualty nurse examined him and telephoned the doctor. The doctor refused to see Mr Barnett, made a diagnosis over the telephone and promptly told the nurse to send him home. Mr Barnett died later from arsenic poisoning. The court judged that the hospital had assumed a duty of care by admitting the patient at the start and therefore the doctor owed him a duty of care. By refusing to see the man he had acted negligently. However, if a hospital closes its accident and emergency department there can be no liability if a patient suffers damage whilst being taken elsewhere because no relationship ever existed between hospital and patient.

2. Breach of duty – proving negligence

The patient bears the burden of proving negligence. He must prove on the balance of probabilities (that it was more likely than not) that the nurse was negligent. The standard of skill and care expected of a nurse is that of the reasonable nurse in the circumstances of the defendant. In order to establish nursing negligence it must be shown that the nurse acted contrary to good professional practice; that she did, or did not do, something which no reasonable nurse would do, or fail to do. An instructive case on this issue is *Wilsher* v. *Essex AHA* (1986). Martin Wilsher was born in 1978 three months prematurely. Martin was placed in an incubator and given extra oxygen. A catheter was inserted into a vein instead of an artery thereby giving incorrect readings of oxygen levels in the baby's blood. The junior doctor who inserted the catheter asked the registrar, who was also relatively inexperienced, to look at Martin. The registrar failed to notice the mistake with the result that Martin received excess oxygen for twelve hours and later developed retrolental fibroplasia. The Court of Appeal decided that the junior house officer had acted reasonably in realising that something was wrong and calling his senior. The registrar, however, had failed to exercise the skill of a reasonable registrar. The court recognised that he had done his best and that he lacked the necessary experience and training for the very specialised care Martin needed. Nonetheless he was held negligent.

There is a stigma attached to the word 'negligence'. Health professionals may feel that it is a moral condemnation of their behaviour or some form of punishment. In law, negligence does not always equate to incompetence. Unlike most other professionals, health professionals often do not get a chance to rectify their mistakes and their mistakes often have serious consequences. But remember, establishing negligence may be the only way for the patient to get compensation for his injury.

The standard of care demanded of a nurse is thus the standard of the reasonably skilled and experienced nurse in the defendant's speciality:

> The test is the standard of the ordinary skilled [person] exercising or professing to have that special skill. A [person] need not possess the highest expert skill; it is well established law that it is sufficient if he exercises the ordinary skill of an ordinary competent [person] exercising that particular art. (*Bolam* v. *Friern HMC* (1957) p. 586)

So in trying to establish a breach of duty the question to be asked first is: has the nurse attained the required standard of care? In Chapter Four you were introduced to the concept of accepted medical practice established in *Bolam*. The test asserts that as long as a doctor acts:

> in accordance with a practice accepted as proper by a responsible body of medical men skilled in that particular area . . . a man is not negligent, if he is acting in accordance with such a practice, merely because there is a body of opinion who would take a contrary view. (pp. 587–8)

Although the test is couched in medical terms it is a universal test for all professionals. The case of *Whitehouse* v. *Jordan* (1981) provides a good example of the accepted practice test. Mrs Whitehouse was a very petite woman suffering an extremely difficult labour. The attending doctor summoned the senior registrar, Mr Jordan, who attempted to deliver the baby by forceps. After pulling six times without success he moved on to deliver the child by Caesarean section. The baby was severely brain damaged. Mrs Whitehouse claimed that the damage was caused by the excessive force used in the trial of forceps. The House of Lords found Mr Jordan not liable in negligence because he was able to provide expert evidence that he had acted in accordance with a body of accepted professional opinion – other doctors attested that in similar circumstances they would have acted in the same way. It made no difference that the plaintiff also provided expert witnesses who testified that they would have acted completely differently.

Where there is conflicting expert evidence it matters not how eminent the plaintiff's witnesses are. The courts will not choose between conflicting expert evidence as the following decision illustrates. In *Maynard* v. *West Midlands RHA* (1984), Mrs Maynard complained of symptoms common to tuberculosis and Hodgkin's disease. Both the consultant physician and the surgeon she approached decided that a mediastinoscopy should be performed to discover which of the conditions Mrs Maynard was actually suffering from. This diagnostic operation carries a risk of damage to the vocal cords and that damage did in fact occur. Mrs Maynard proved to have tuberculosis. She complained that the doctors were negligent in subjecting her to the mediastinoscopy when her circumstances indicated that it was more likely than not that she was suffering from tuberculosis. The defendants argued that the fatality rate for Hodgkin's disease if treatment were delayed justified them in exposing Mrs Maynard to the risk of the mediastinoscopy. The judge at first instance preferred the plaintiff's expert's evidence. The Court of Appeal and the House of Lords overruled his decision and said: '. . . a judge's preference for one body of distinguished professional opinion to another also professionally distinguished is not sufficient to establish negligence in a practitioner' (p. 639).

To date then, in England the health professional is highly unlikely to be found liable in negligence if she acts in conformity with a practice accepted by at least a respectable number of her peers. The courts have said that there might, in theory, be examples of a professional practice so clearly irreconcilable with the duty owed to a patient, that a judge would find it to be negligent despite its endorsement by professionals themselves. But no English court has yet ever thus condemned a practice endorsed by medical or nursing opinion. Everything turns on the expert evidence. The burden of proving negligence for a patient-plaintiff is thus heavy indeed.

Departing from standard practice

But what if the nurse departs from standard practice? Is she then likely to be found negligent? Legal principles that found any departure from standard practice resulting in injury to be negligent would stifle innovation and reduce nursing to blind obedience to sets of rules and regulations. The position now is this. Even where a patient can prove the nurse did not conform to accepted practice, it is still up to him to show that her treatment of him was negligent. However, if the nurse cannot produce evidence to explain and justify her unconventional treatment of the patient, the patient is likely to succeed in his claim. Nurses must not be afraid to exercise initiative; they must ensure that they can justify their actions.

Diagnosis and treatment

Nurses in 1994 find themselves required to take responsibility for a greater independent role in diagnosis and treatment. How far does enhanced independence place the nurse at greater risk of legal liability?

A wrong diagnosis is not, on its own, evidence of negligence on the part of any health professional. As the case of *Hunter* v. *Hanley* (1955) indicates, 'there is ample scope for a genuine difference of opinion and one man is clearly not negligent merely because his conclusion differs from that of other professional men' (p. 217).

In order to establish that a wrong diagnosis was negligent the plaintiff must show that the professional failed to carry out an examination or test which the symptoms called for or that the eventual conclusion was one that no reasonable professional would have come to. Again, expert evidence is crucial. Negligence is more easily found when there has been a specific failure, i.e. to act on information available or to perform routine tests. Nurses should actively seek information from patients; never rely entirely on information supplied by colleagues; check dosages – readily prescribing an overdose amounts to negligence; and read drug labelling carefully and properly. In *Sutton* v. *Population Services* (1981) a nurse working in a Family Planning Clinic, who did not note or did not act on evidence of a lump in a patient's breast, was held to be negligent. The reasonable nurse would have taken steps to investigate the lump which ultimately proved to be cancerous.

The more independent the nurse's role or function, the more likely it is that he will be held personally responsible. Where he has responsibility for diagnosis and choice of treatment his responsibility equates with that of medical team members. Treatment may be negligent either by choosing inappropriate treatment or by carrying out the correct treatment carelessly. In the former case the test will be whether the chosen method of treatment conformed with accepted practice. To avoid liability for negligent performance of the treatment the nurse must once again act on adequate information; be alert to common drug reactions and communicate effectively with patients. He must ensure that he is fully up-to-date with developments in current practice. The law will readily condemn the nurse who fails in his ethical obligations to maintain his competence and expertise. He must be meticulous in carrying out every task. Particular care must be taken in administering drugs, as using the wrong drug or administering an overdose will rarely be excused. The nurse must not rely blindly on what he thinks a doctor requires. In *Prendergrast* v. *Dee* (1989) a doctor's handwriting was so atrocious that the pharmacist dispensed the wrong drug with disastrous consequences. The doctor was found negligent for his careless means of communicating with the pharmacist. The pharmacist was negligent in failing to exercise his judgment and recognise the clearly inappropriate nature of the drug which he thought that the doctor had prescribed. Do not rely on a doctor's scrawl. Do not accept unquestioningly an instruction from a weary junior doctor which your professional instinct tells you is wrong.

Effective treatment is very much concerned with team work and joint responsibility. Within a team a nurse may be liable in negligence if he fails to take proper notice of instructions or fails to provide adequate care or attention. In *Smith* v. *Brighton and Lewes HMC* (1955) a patient was prescribed thirty injections of streptomycin for boils. The sister did not record on the notes when the course was completed. Four extra injections were given before the error was discovered and the patient suffered damage to the cranial nerve. The sister was found to be negligent. Liability for negligence will often be apportioned between doctors and nurses working together. For example, in the operating theatre both surgeons and theatre sisters are responsible for checking that all instruments and swabs have been removed. If anything is left behind both may be held legally accountable for the failure.

Inexperience, junior staff and overwork

Very often nurses who do make negligent mistakes do so either because they find themselves forced to undertake tasks beyond their experience, or because long hours at work and inadequate resources leave them exhausted. The overtired nurse may well be morally blameless but where legal accountability is concerned no allowance is made for inexperience, overtiredness or overwork. In *Nettleship* v. *Weston* (1971) a learner driver was held liable for injuries sustained by her instructor. Although she had done her incompetent best, she had failed to attain the standard of the reasonably competent and experienced motorist. The fact that nurses are made to work to the point where exhaustion impairs judgment and ability will not affect the patient's claim for negligence. The overtired nurse will remain accountable and liable to the patient.

The junior nurse 'forced' to carry out a task which she feels that she is not yet qualified to do remains legally responsible for her patient. In *Wilsher* v. *Essex AHA* neither the senior house officer or the registrar should have been left alone in charge of the unit. Their counsel argued that the doctors should be judged not by the standard to be expected of a reasonably qualified and experienced person in charge of such a unit, but in the light of the doctors' actual experience and training. The Court of Appeal rejected the argument. You are legally responsible for the tasks you undertake. If they are beyond your competence you must seek help or refuse to carry on. That advice is easier said than done. The rigidity of the legal rules is ameliorated somewhat by the fact that, in reality, the nurse is unlikely to be sued personally. The patient will sue her employer, the NHS trust or health authority. Even if a patient insists on suing the nurse as well, NHS indemnity rules ensure that her employer must normally meet her legal costs and any award made against her.

3. Causation

Even if negligence on the part of a nurse is clearly proven, for a law suit to succeed, the patient must show that his injury was caused or aggravated by the nurse's acts or omissions. Sometimes establishing the link between act and injury is easy because had it not been for the negligent performance of the treatment, the plaintiff would never have suffered any injury; for example, where a swab is left in the patient's abdomen after surgery. Many claims, however, are not usually so straightforward. A number of factors may contribute to a particular outcome, not least of which may be the illness or injury itself. If the patient cannot prove that the relevant negligence actually caused his injury he will fail. Reflect on the case of Martin Wilsher. The court held that there had been negligence but ultimately Martin still failed to get compensation. It could not be established that the negligence, the administration of excess oxygen, caused his blindness. Scientific evidence indicated that although excess oxygen may cause retrolental fibroplasia there were five other possible causes of that condition in very premature and sick babies. Hence, wherever there is more than one cause, the plaintiff's claim may well be doomed to failure. The quality of the patient's scientific evidence and expert witnesses is crucial.

There is no greater prospect of success where the evidence shows that, had the patient been treated properly, there was only a chance that he would have escaped the injury. In *Hotson* v. *East Berkshire AHA* (1987) the plaintiff argued that he had been denied a 25 per cent chance of full recovery. At the age of thirteen he had an accident which left him permanently disabled. He injured his hip in a fall but on arrival at the hospital the injury was not diagnosed and he was sent home. Five days later, and still in pain, he returned to hospital whereupon the extent of his injuries was discovered and he was treated immediately. The health authority admitted negligence in respect of the delayed diagnosis but denied that the resulting delay had impaired the plaintiff's long-term condition. On the expert evidence given, the trial judge found that even if the condition had been correctly diagnosed and promptly treated there was a 75 per cent chance that the plaintiff's disability would develop anyway, but that the medical staff's breach of duty had turned that risk into an inevitability. The plaintiff lost a 25 per cent chance of a full recovery, and the trial judge awarded him compensation for that lost chance.

In the House of Lords the central issue was whether the plaintiff's injury was caused by his fall or by the authority's negligence in making an incorrect diagnosis and delaying treatment. The Lords decided that the plaintiff's injuries on arrival at the hospital on the first occasion were such that even had his condition been correctly diagnosed and treated there was a 75 per cent probability that the disability would have occurred anyway. The plaintiff had failed to prove that the negligent delay had in fact caused his disability. He had not proved it was more likely than not that the defendants' negligence resulted in that long-term disability. His damages were limited to compensation for pain and suffering over five days only.

Suing for nursing negligence

If the preceding pages terrify you, never forget that in practice claims against nurses are rare. In all forms of health care litigation the dice are in fact loaded against the patient. Legal aid is available only to the very poor and tremendous financial hurdles face patients who want to sue. They may need a court order to obtain access to crucial medical records. The right of access to health records applies only to records compiled after November 1991. Health care litigation is complex and may take years to resolve. Martin Wilsher was ten before his case reached the House of Lords.

The law ultimately defines the nurse's responsibility to care for patients. But it does and can do no more than set the basic standard every nurse must meet. The tort of negligence acts as a deterrent against doing harm – non-maleficence – it does not actively promote doing good – beneficence. The practical difficulties of litigation mean additionally that perhaps the law is not even a very effective deterrent. Yet more and more patients are resorting to litigation. It should not be thought that their motives are always financial. Many plaintiff-patients see litigation as the only means of finding out what went wrong with treatment and holding the responsible professional accountable for their actions. As we have noted, for the present, a nurse is unlikely to be named personally in a lawsuit and in any case her employer will indemnify her against both costs and damages if she is sued. The nurse's accountability is more likely to be enforced before the Professional Conduct Committee of the UKCC or in disciplinary proceedings instituted by her employer. Before looking at those sorts of proceedings, though, we should return again to the implications of an extended scope of nursing practice role, for the more the patient perceives the nurse as an independent professional the more likely it is that legal proceedings will be taken against her personally.

The 'extended role' and the independent nurse practitioner

Titles such as 'extended role' and 'independent nurse practitioner' have been used to describe developments which result in nurses taking on greater responsibility and performing tasks which have traditionally been considered as belonging to the medical profession. A few examples of this include diagnosis and treatment of minor acute illnesses; basic prescriptions for dressings and ointments; administration of intravenous drugs; cervical smears and ear syringing.

Many nurses have been apprehensive about taking on an 'extended role' because they fear that they will open themselves up to legal liability. To combat these fears, from time to time, various procedures were developed to 'certify' the nurse's competence to take on an extended role and to provide 'legitimate' authority for such acceptance. However, it is generally considered today that the concept of the 'extended role' is no longer appropriate and that, rather than extending or enhancing nursing practice, the terminology may limit the role of nurses. As medical technology advances, nurses will continue to adopt new practices and techniques – this in itself is a role of nursing. Certification is no longer seen to be appropriate or necessary.

The extent of the nurse's role and responsibilities is now guided by the UKCC document entitled *The Scope of Professional Practice* (1992). This document provides a framework for practice which emphasises the personal responsibility and accountability of individual professionals for their own practice, development and maintenance of their knowledge and competence. They must be guided by the UKCC *Code of Professional Conduct* and other advisory documents.

As far as the law is concerned, the continually expanding role of the nurse raises no new issues. A certificate has never provided blanket immunity from legal liability. If a competent nurse accepted a role without proper authorisation, the law was only concerned if she harmed a patient through her negligence. What matters if an action is brought for negligence is simply whether, in the performance of the task which she has undertaken, the nurse achieves the level of competence which that task demands. What constitutes that level of competence will be judged by her peers. A nurse who takes on responsibilities for which she knows she is not trained or competent may be liable in negligence if, through her inexperience or incompetence, she causes a patient harm. The primary role of the nurse in whatever capacity is to be aware of her responsibilities towards her patients and to be able to account for her actions.

Accountability – outside the courtroom

The nurse who falls below the required professional standard will in nine out of ten instances find herself called to account not in a court of law but before the UKCC or her employer. Her conduct may also be investigated by the NHS Ombudsman. In any of these cases what this will entail is an investigation of how the nurse behaved. The outcome of any error, whether or not it resulted in any actual injury, will not be relevant.

Professional discipline – the UKCC

When an allegation of professional misconduct is made to the UKCC against a nurse, whether by managers, colleagues, patients, or by notification of a criminal conviction, the complaint must be investigated. The UKCC has a statutory responsibility to investigate all complaints and to ensure that the complainant has her case fully heard and must allow the nurse in question to defend herself. If the allegation is found to have sufficient grounds after examination of written statements, the Professional Conduct Committee (PCC) holds a public hearing in which it decides whether the charges are proved and the incident did occur. A decision is then made as to whether the nurse's conduct amounts to professional misconduct.

Most allegations of misconduct arise from mistakes at work. The following example is a case which came before the PCC. At the end of a hectic day in theatre, the operating theatre sister responsible for checking the instruments left for home having left the instruments in the washer. The following day she was informed by two night staff that a pair of forceps was missing from the abdominal set. The regulations stated that if a replacement instrument was needed the senior manager must be informed. Concerned about the day ahead, the theatre sister did not want to make a fuss and helped herself to a spare pair of forceps. Two weeks later the elderly gentleman who had been the last patient in theatre that night died unexpectedly. The autopsy revealed the missing pair of forceps lodged in the man's abdomen. The nurse was dismissed immediately and the matter referred to the UKCC. The allegation was that she had acted irresponsibly when the instrument was reported missing and acted inappropriately to conceal the incident – a breach of clause two. At the hearing the nurse argued that the fault lay with the hospital standard practice of leaving responsibility for checks with one person.

Genuine mistakes made in the emergency of a situation will normally be viewed sympathetically by the UKCC, but in this case it was the dishonesty of the nurse's actions in hiding the error that troubled the Committee. Judgment was postponed for three months and the nurse was asked to supply a reference from her new employer which had to be written with knowledge of the incident.

If a nurse is found guilty of professional misconduct the Professional Conduct Committee of the UKCC may take a number of actions as follows:

1. Judgment may be postponed in order to take references and additional reports.
2. Referral may be made to the health committee which deals with nurses who are unsafe to practise due to illness rather than misconduct – usually a nurse will be reinstated when she can prove that she is no longer unsafe to practise.
3. The nurse may be suspended.
4. She may be cautioned.
5. She may be removed from the register.

No hard and fast rules can be identified as each case depends a great deal, not only on the nurse's conduct, but on her character, previous conduct and references, and the background to the event (including managerial and hospital administration).

Removal from the register is the ultimate sanction and causes the nurse, amongst other things, loss of livelihood. To ameliorate the severity of the sanction the nurse has two possible courses of action.

1. She may appeal to the High Court – but the court rarely interferes with decisions of the UKCC.
2. She may apply for restoration to the register after twelve to eighteen months. The nurse must prove to the Committee that she is worthy of being restored with employer's references, personal testimonials and by demonstrating that the lesson has been learnt.

Hospital complaints procedures and the NHS Ombudsman

The Hospital Complaints Procedures Act 1985 ensures that each hospital provides arrangements for dealing with patients' complaints. A designated officer (often the Unit General Manager) has a duty to receive and handle complaints. Initially all complaints go to him and where the complainant is in agreement he will make attempts at informal conciliation. Where there is no agreement, further action depends on the nature and seriousness of the complaint. The designated officer investigates and acts on minor complaints. More serious complaints must be brought to the attention of senior officers of the authority such as the District General Manager and, where appropriate, the Regional Medical Officer. More serious complaints are classed as follows:

1. A complaint that raises any question of clinical judgment that cannot be resolved by discussion with the consultant concerned.
2. A complaint that the authority is satisfied constitutes a serious unto-ward incident involving harm to a patient.
3. A complaint that involves conduct which ought to be the subject of disciplinary proceedings.
4. A complaint that concerns a possible criminal offence.
5. A complaint that involves the designated officer.

So a complaint against a nurse by a patient about her rudeness and general unhelpfulness will probably be dealt with by the designated hospital officer. On the other hand, a case of a nurse who, through overwork, coped badly on an understaffed maternity ward one night causing delayed treatment and harm to a patient would most likely be considered by senior officers and possibly the Health Service Commissioner.

Where a patient is unhappy with the hospital officer's response to his complaint he may take the matter to the Health Service Commissioner who is known as the NHS Ombudsman. The Commissioner investigates written complaints which allege that a failure or bad administration has caused injustice or hardship; such investigation will include nursing management and all concerned along with the individuals. There are two important limitations on his powers. If the patient concerned may have a remedy in the courts, the Commissioner may not pursue the complaint unless he is satisfied that it would be unreasonable to expect the patient to pursue that remedy. The Commissioner may not investigate any action which is taken by doctors or nurses as a result of exercising their professional or clinical judgment.

If the Commissioner decides that the complaint is justified, an apology will be given. Complaints may be taken further to the regional health authority for investigation and in more serious cases, an independent inquiry can be set up. Ultimately, where the complaint is most serious and much publicised the Health Minister may hold an inquiry – a recent example of which was the case of Beverly Allitt who killed four children while suffering from a psychiatric disorder. Ms Allitt herself was sentenced in the criminal courts but public outrage demanded that the health authority concerned be held to account for the situation arising in the first place.

The point of the Hospital Complaints Procedure is primarily to provide the patient with a procedure to lodge complaints and not to discipline individuals. It might be that at the end of the investigation one or more individuals will be dismissed but that course of action will be taken by the professional's employer.

The health authority and disciplinary action

The disciplinary action taken by a nurse's employer will depend on the nature and severity of the offence and can be anything from a verbal warning to immediate dismissal. Gross misconduct, such as working under the influence of drugs or theft of hospital or patients' property, will often lead to summary dismissal. But more often gross misconduct will result in the nurse being suspended with pay in order to allow a full investigation and for managerial consultation before taking any action. Consider the following example. A Registered Nurse for the Mentally Handicapped was given responsibility for eight patients on a seaside holiday. He was suspended on full pay for obtaining prescriptions from a local GP rather than calling his hospital when he discovered that some 'as required' medicines were missing from the medicine box and for withholding medicines which, in his professional opinion, were inappropriate at the time. No patients complained and it was generally felt that they benefited greatly from the holiday under his supervision. After a full investigation the nurse was dismissed.

Some behaviour, though not gross misconduct, is serious enough to warrant formal disciplinary procedures without an initial informal warning.

This will normally result in a formal verbal warning after a meeting in which the nurse must account for her behaviour. Where facts are clear, a written warning may follow.

Where disciplinary action is taken the nurse may appeal within the health district: first to the appropriate member of the district management team; then to a district health authority appeal committee; and then finally to the regional health authority at the authority's discretion. If insured, the nurse may engage a solicitor to sue the authority. The third possibility is for her to go to an industrial tribunal claiming unfair or wrongful dismissal. If the tribunal finds that the nurse has been unfairly dismissed it may recommend that the nurse be re-employed or re-instated but cannot enforce that recommendation.

Natural justice – the role of the law

Wherever a governing body is in a position to decide on the actions of an individual, the principles of natural justice will apply. In the case where a nurse is removed from the register by the UKCC or is dismissed by her employers and she appeals to the High Court, the court will judge the actions of the body in accordance with the rules of natural justice. The rules of natural justice are the most basic standards of fair decision-making. They provide that no person shall be judge in his own cause and that each party must be given a fair hearing. The first rule demands that the adjudicator must have no bias. The second rule has two limbs. No person may be penalised by a decision of an adjudicating body unless she has been given (1) prior notice of the charge to be met, and (2) a fair opportunity to answer the case against her and to put forward her own case. The purpose of the rules is to ensure that where an accusation is made, the accused has a right to be heard and to defend herself.

The concept of natural justice is important as a way in which a court may supervise and regulate the fairness of proceedings of the UKCC and any other adjudicating body. If the court feels that a decision has been made in contravention of natural justice it may intervene and reverse the decision (although this is rarely the outcome). The court's role is therefore to assess the procedural fairness of the hearing rather than to 'retry' the case on its facts. The case of *Hefferen* v. *the Committee of the UKCC* (1988) is a rare example of court intervention. Hefferen was a community nurse specialising in baby care. On one hurried occasion she gave a child the wrong injection but then realised her mistake and reported it to the doctor. She told the mother and also made a record in the child's notes. What she failed to do was to write to the health visitor and sister in charge of the clinic. When they discovered the error they informed the health authority and Hefferen was summarily dismissed. She was subsequently removed from the register for that failure. The court found, when she appealed, that the procedure followed by the Conduct Committee was unfair and reversed the decision. A change in the UKCC rules brought in new allegations at a later stage in the action against Hefferen, thereby preventing her from defending her case adequately. In other situations the court may decide to send the case back to the UKCC for the facts to be heard and decided on again.

Conclusion

Legal and professional duties share a common language encompassing concepts of responsibility and accountability, yet the way in which the nurse may be held to account may differ enormously. In practice the nurse will face ethical dilemmas continually and the purpose here is to provide some guidance as to how those dilemmas might be approached. Legal accountability is much less common for nurses. If a nurse appears in court at all she will usually be there as a witness giving evidence – nevertheless she remains accountable. Whether or not a nurse is ever held to account for her actions, her choices should be determined by her ethical and legal responsibilities. The Code provides the basis for ethical conduct and there-fore good professional practice. In law the responsibility is to act in ac-cordance with accepted practice and it would appear that professional practice, as prescribed by the UKCC, will influence accepted practice and therefore legal liability.

8

Pregnancy and childbirth

Ethical and legal problems encountered in caring for patients generally are compounded when your patient is a pregnant woman. Instead of just one patient whose interests you must respect, you arguably now have two patients, the woman and her unborn child. The interests of mother and child will not always coincide. In their most dramatic context maternal/foetal conflicts of interest require you to consider whether respect for the autonomy of the pregnant woman permits her to terminate the existence of the foetus. And, if your answer is yes, are you required to assist in that act? Does the stage of foetal development, when the woman seeks an induced abortion, matter? What should happen if a woman goes to full term but in the course of labour rejects an intervention that you, the professional, consider necessary to preserve the life of the child? More routine incidences of maternal/foetal conflict of interest include what should be done when a pregnant woman suffers from acute sickness or needs a general anaesthetic in pregnancy. Doing what is best for the mother may endanger the child.

At the heart of all these ethical dilemmas are these fundamental questions. What is the moral and legal status of the unborn child? Can an entity have rights prior to birth? When does life begin?

Ethical considerations

There are differing claims about when human life comes into existence and these different interpretations are often thought relevant to the question of deciding what status should be afforded to the human embryo. What status the human embryo has is in turn important for the debate on abortion and embryo research. Whether an embryo can be killed is dependent upon the status it is given.

From conception

The claim that human life exists from the moment of conception seems plausible. The sperm and the ovum both contain twenty-three chromosomes, and fertilisation of the ovum by the sperm causes the creation of a new individual. This is essentially a biological definition, but is also used as a theological basis for the beginning of life when associated with the infusion of the soul into the embryo by God. However, the early Christian Church did not always agree exactly when ensoulment took place. Knowing nothing of the actual biological process of fertilisation Augustine thought that quickening, that is, the first foetal movements felt by the mother, was the point at which ensoulment took place. Aquinas decided upon forty days after conception for males and eighty days for females.

Acceptance of any religious thesis that life begins at conception will depend upon personal beliefs, but leaving this aside, even the biological definition is not straightforward. Following fertilisation, instead of normal embryonic development, a hydatidiform mole (a growth threatening the life of the mother) may develop. This condition, although relatively rare, occurs in early pregnancy and results from an abnormal development of placental tissue. No embryo ever exists. If human life is considered to begin at conception, then difficulties arise with the hydatidiform mole as it would clearly be absurd to suggest that that growth was a new individual to be given the same respect as any other person, yet it results from the process of fertilisation. And there is another difficulty with this biological argument. Sperm and ova are as much alive as any resulting embryo.

The potentiality argument

Perhaps an alternative approach is to argue that fertilisation is crucial because even though the fertilised ovum is not yet identical to you and me, it has the potential to become so. While this may be true, it does not follow that because the fertilised ovum has the potential to become an adult we should treat it as though it already were. You may have the potential to earn an annual salary of £100,000 in the future, but we doubt that anyone would suggest that this would be a good reason for you to be paid that salary now. Another difficulty with this argument is the fact that the ovum and sperm also enjoy the potential to become a human being. This is, of course, dependent upon the right conditions for fertilisation but then the embryo, foetus, baby and child are all dependent upon the right conditions to allow them to actualise their potential for becoming an adult. Must the ovum and sperm therefore also be given the same respect as an adult? This would be practically difficult, if not impossible to achieve. John Harris in *The Value of Life* contends that the potentiality argument logically requires us to act to ensure each ovum and sperm enjoys the best possible chance of fulfilling its potential. That means no contraception and a moral duty to engage in procreative sexual intercourse as often as possible!

When does life matter?

Perhaps instead of trying to fix a point when human life begins we should
ask a rather different question: why and when does human life matter?
Sperm, ova, embryo, child and adult are all biologically forms of human
life. Yet hardly any of us have problems with the regular destruction of
ova lost in the menstrual flow or the 'loss' of millions of sperm. For those
whose belief system rejects any concept of ensoulment and/or acceptance
of a divine purpose in the creation of humanity, two arguments may have
particular relevance in deciding when human life matters.

First, there is the issue of sentience, the ability to feel pain or pleasure.
The fertilised ovum, the newly formed embryo cannot feel pain, cannot be
hurt by its destruction. Once sentience exists then you might argue the
foetus should not be hurt any more than any other sentient being should
be harmed. Arguments based on sentience obviously relate not just to
embryos but also to any other non-sentient human being such as the
patient in a permanent vegetative state. Moral arguments based on sentience legitimate early abortion and embryo research. However, sentience
is not an argument that takes you all that far. It prohibits only hurting the
sentient entity. It would require that any method of abortion avoid such
hurt, but does not offer any absolute protection to the foetus. We consider
it unethical to hurt animals and have laws to prevent cruelty, but we do
not ban the killing of animals. So how are humans different? Moral philosophers such as Singer and Harris argue that what is crucial is not
whether an entity is a member of the human species but whether he or she
is a human person. What distinguishes you from your pet cat is simply
this. You are able to value your own existence, to recollect what you did
yesterday and plan what you will do tomorrow. The foetus lacks that
capacity at any stage of its journey to birth and, indeed, the newborn
infant similarly lacks that capacity. They are not yet persons and so cannot
claim moral rights of their own.

There is a less radical version of the above argument that in a sense links
sentience and personhood. It is the inherent nature of the human brain
that creates the capacity to reason and to value existence. Lockwood among
others argues, then, that at the stage of foetal development (about eight to
ten weeks) when electrical activity in the brain is first discernible, when brain
life begins, the foetus acquires an independent moral status. Just as brain
stem death is diagnosed by the cessation of such activity, so the inception
of brain activity should mark the point when life begins to matter.

This brief discussion of the diversity of opinion on the status of the
unborn child illustrates the profound difficulty the care of the pregnant
woman poses for any nurse. For once you decide the embryo or foetus has
moral rights of its own, those rights create the potential of conflict with
the rights of its mother.

Abortion

The disputed moral status of the foetus then makes it scarcely surprising that abortion is one of the most widely discussed and problematic issues in the subject of health care ethics and that there have been many papers and books written about the subject. Even twenty-five years after the Abortion Act passed through Parliament, debate continues and there are no signs of a decrease in interest in this subject. Moreover, the abortion debate continues to generate passion to the extent that in the USA 'pro-life' groups have physically attacked health professionals involved in abortion, and one doctor has even been killed by an assailant who branded the doctor as a 'murderer'. Abortion raises complex issues which relate back, of course, in many instances to the status of the foetus. But the status of the foetus is not the only relevant issue. Even if you regard the foetus as having independent moral rights, the mother too has equivalent rights. You cannot conclude that just because the foetus has moral claims, those claims should take priority over those of the mother. We cannot possibly canvass all the pertinent arguments in the abortion debate. So let us look primarily at the conflict between what could be broadly regarded as the conservative and the liberal views of abortion.

The conservative view

People holding the conservative view usually oppose abortion because of the status they afford to the foetus. A conservative argument would state that killing innocent human beings is wrong. The foetus is an innocent human being, and therefore killing the foetus is also wrong. The development of the fertilised ovum into the embryo, and then into the foetus, and finally the baby is seen as a gradual process with no clear dividing line between one stage and the next. Because of this gradual process it is not possible to show any morally significant point when an abortion may be performed. Therefore, we must grant the fertilised ovum the same moral status as that of a baby because there is no significant point when we can distinguish between one and the other. The ultra-conservative would not consider abortion morally permissible in any circumstances at any stage of pregnancy. The innocent life of the foetus takes priority over any interests of the mother, even her life and health.

The conservative view is most closely identified with the official teaching of the Roman Catholic Church. But it is a view shared by a number of non-Catholic Christians too, particularly evangelical Protestants. As life begins at conception, then the foetus has the same right to life as any other individual. One of the difficulties with the conservative view is the extent to which it depends on a theological justification. We live in a largely secular society. Even among those who profess a faith, the conservative approach to abortion is not universal. Neither Islam nor Judaism has ever outlawed abortion completely. Both religions regard the foetus as having moral significance but consider that there are circumstances where the mother must be accorded greater significance. Conservative arguments based on biology run into the problems discussed earlier that there truly is no definitive point when life begins.

The 'easy' answer to the conservative argument is this. It binds only those who believe in it. So for one of the authors of this book who accepts that her religion mandates that she regard any embryo as morally equivalent to herself, abortion is not an option. But she has no right to enforce that belief on others. The 'easy' answer has, alas, an inherent flaw. Assuming the majority of the population decided redheads were not human beings, that would not immediately make it right for those who held that belief to go ahead and kill any passing redhead. Belief that the embryo is morally equivalent to any adult human necessarily renders any destruction of the embryo morally equivalent to murder in the eyes of those who maintain that view.

The liberal view

Those who hold a liberal view of abortion may do so on two main grounds. They may reject claims that the foetus has any moral status. It may be of human origin but it is not a person. It follows then that there are no grounds to interfere with the mother's right to manage her pregnancy and labour as she chooses, nor to prevent her destroying the foetus. Alternatively it might be argued that yes, the foetus does enjoy moral status and rights but any such rights are always subordinate to those of the mother. The foetus is a part of her body; she retains absolute control over her body. This argument, often associated with feminism, also renders unjustifiable any restrictions on access to abortion. However, because moral status is accorded to the foetus, albeit a status subordinated to the mother's, the foetus can have rights against third parties. It has a legitimate claim not to be injured *in utero* by, for example, teratogenic drugs.

The ultra-liberal view, whatever its philosophical basis, requires that abortion be freely available on demand at any stage in pregnancy. If a woman seeks abortion at thirty-six weeks gestation in order not to lose the opportunity to climb Everest, there are no sufficient reasons to deny her that choice. Put as starkly as that, many who reject the conservative stance on abortion may find they also have problems with the liberal approach.

Abortion as a continuum

The conservative and liberal camps both have their vehement supporters. Realistically, though, many others probably view the abortion debate as a continuum with the extreme conservative and liberal views at opposite poles. In between the two poles you find several more moderate viewpoints. Some people, for example, tending to a conservative view, may consider abortion permissible in certain clearly defined circumstances such as pregnancy as a result of rape. Others with a liberal attitude, although agreeing with abortion in principle, may want to set a time limit for abortions to be carried out. They would not consider it permissible to carry out abortions in the final weeks of pregnancy. Other individuals may not agree with abortion except on grounds of substantial risk to the health of the mother or foetal abnormality.

But 'moderate' arguments can become rather complex and often difficult to sustain because if someone believes that the foetus has the same right to life as an adult, then how the pregnancy occurred is not relevant to the status of that foetus. Someone arguing that abortion should be allowed in cases of rape only would need to identify what was different about the status of the foetus in this particular case. In a similar way, if you believe that the foetus is part of the woman's body and not afforded rights of its own, then what grounds would you have for arguing that an abortion should not be carried out after a certain gestation period or even just because the woman wants to climb Everest?

The consequentialist view

A consequentialist might argue that instead of trying to decide if the foetus has a right to life or if the woman has a right to do what she wants with her body, we should consider the consequences of performing or not performing an abortion. After all, the debate on those questions appears never-ending. In general the consequentialist will support a liberal view of abortion and yet accept that the foetus has human status. The interests of the woman, the foetus, other members of the family and society in general need to be considered in turn so that a decision can be made which will maximise the satisfaction of these interests. For example, a consequentialist may argue that it is better for society if a liberal abortion policy exists as women will seek illegal abortions if the facility is not available. The 1967 Abortion Act brought a dramatic decrease in the number of maternal deaths attributed to abortion which is obviously of benefit to society, and, although abortions will cause the death of foetuses, they prevent women dying at the hands of illegal abortionists. In the same way, the consequentialist may decide that abortion on the grounds of foetal abnormality should be allowed. The interests of the woman, her partner and other children may only be satisfied if they do not have a disabled baby and these together would outweigh the interests of the foetus. The consequentialist is likely to be lambasted as unsound by both conservative and liberal camps.

Caring for women having abortions

Were you not a student nurse, all the abortion debate would demand of you is that you settle your own stance on abortion. You would have to decide where on the continuum you find your place. However, as a nurse you may find yourself asked to participate in an abortion in circumstances which contravene your own moral code. Have you the right to refuse to take part?

The Abortion Act 1967 contains what is termed a conscience clause which states that health professionals have a right to refuse to participate in any treatment authorised by the Act. This is usually interpreted by nurses to mean that they may refuse to play any part or be present when an abortion is being performed in either the operating theatre or any other clinical area where the procedure may be undertaken. Clause eight of the *Code of Professional Conduct* recognises this right, but states that nurses must make conscientious objections known at the earliest possible time. Nurses do not have the option to refuse to participate in the care of such women at any other time such as pre- or post-operatively. The right of conscientious objection is limited to a right to withdraw from any direct involvement in the destruction of the foetus. Furthermore, it must be forsaken in an emergency situation where the mother's life is threatened or where it is necessary to intervene to prevent grave injury to her health.

Should nurses be allowed to opt out of abortions at all? It could be argued that nurses refusing to participate in the care of women undergoing abortions are not fulfilling their professional role as they should care for all patients and clients irrespective of the services they require. A nurse could not, for example, refuse to care for an alcoholic patient because her own moral code or religion condemned alcohol abuse. While all patients and clients should be treated with the same amount of care irrespective of their needs, the problem of abortion is quite different from any other ethical issue in health care. Abortion causes the destruction of a foetus, and while some will argue that there are circumstances when this is both legally and morally the right action to take, others do equate abortion with murder. There would be nothing to gain by forcing nurses to participate in abortions against their will, especially as this could be detrimental to the care of women requiring this service. As a consequence, the most practical solution for both health professionals and women is to consider abortion a special case.

The law relating to pregnancy and childbirth

The diversity of opinion on the moral status of the foetus makes the role of the law in relation to unborn children exceptionally difficult. If there is no consensus on whether foetuses have rights, legislating on issues such as abortion and embryo research becomes a nightmare. The Abortion Act 1967, as amended by the Human Fertilisation and Embryology Act 1990, represents an attempt at compromise. Before we examine that compromise, however, we need to look more generally at the legal status afforded to the unborn child and see what protection the law affords her or him. The thalidomide tragedy illustrated all too well the vulnerability of the foetus. Thalidomide, marketed as safe for use in pregnancy, was taken by women across the world and resulted in the live birth of children suffering dreadful deformities. If the unborn child receives no legal recognition, then such prenatal injuries cannot be compensated. What duty, if any, is owed to the unborn child?

Congenital Disabilities (Civil Liability) Act 1976

Prior to the enactment of this statute, it was unclear whether English law recognised any duty at all to take care to avoid injuring the foetus. Negligent antenatal care that resulted in the birth of a disabled child might give the mother a right to sue you, but the child's rights were undefined. The Congenital Disabilities (Civil Liability) Act provided that if a child is born alive suffering from a disability resulting from an occurrence which either (a) affected either parent in his or her ability to have healthy children, or (b) affected the mother in pregnancy or (c) affected mother or child in labour, the child may be able to recover compensation for its prenatal injury. But the relevant occurrence must be one which would also give rise to liability to the affected parent. Mothers are generally granted immunity from any action against them on behalf of the child.

The complicated provisions of the 1976 Act mean this in practice. Health professionals are legally required to take care to avoid any measure which might damage a patient's reproductive capacity or damage the foetus *in utero*. Prescribing a drug which you ought to know may cause foetal deformity is legally actionable. The 1976 Act largely avoids any dispute over the moral status of the foetus. The foetal right is a derivative right only, a right to compensation for the damage it suffers as a result of negligent treatment of its parent. No conflict of interest between mother and foetus is created by the Act. First, the foetus, even when born alive, has no rights it can assert against its mother. Second, there has to be a wrong committed against a parent before liability to the child can arise. So if after proper consultation a mother agrees to an anaesthetic when she needs surgery, the child cannot bring a claim if the anaesthetic injures her or him in the womb.

The 1976 Act was designed as a pragmatic piece of legislation to ensure that if a third party injured a child prenatally, the child and the family could obtain proper compensation. It does not work very well because all too often it is impossible to prove the link between the allegedly injurious occurrence and the child's actual disability. A recent case concerned the high incidence of leukaemia in the offspring of men who worked at a nuclear power station. It was claimed that the fathers' sperm had been damaged by exposure to radiation, but the claim failed because there just was not enough evidence of cause and effect. Another problem with the Act is this. It only covers cases where some negligence on the part of the defendant actually causes the child's disability and is limited to wrongful disability claims. A more common scenario in relation to health professionals is that some negligence of theirs, while it does not damage the foetus directly, results in the birth of a child whom the parents would not have wished to be born, or indeed the birth of a child so disabled that the child itself might prefer not to have been born. A common cause of such a wrongful birth or wrongful life claim is that negligent antenatal screening failed to detect abnormalities in the foetus. Had the mother been aware of the foetal abnormality she would have terminated the pregnancy.

Wrongful birth and wrongful life

A wrongful birth claim may be brought whenever parents claim that, but for the negligence of the defendant, no birth would have occurred. One common example of a wrongful birth claim arises out of a failed sterilisation operation. The mother proves either that the gynaecologist bungled the operation or failed to warn her that there is always a risk that the operation will fail and nature will restore fertility. In the latter case she argues that had she known sterilisation was not 100 per cent effective, she would have realised that she was pregnant soon enough to have an early abortion. After some initial reservation, the Court of Appeal in *Emeh* v. *Kensington and Chelsea AHA* (1985) allowed such claims. Another example of a wrongful birth claim resulting in professional liability can be seen in *Salih* v. *Enfield AHA* (1991). The defendants negligently carried out tests for rubella after the mother came into contact with the disease early in pregnancy. The mother was therefore wrongly told that the tests were negative and that the foetus was undamaged. In the event, when the child was born, he suffered from multiple disabilities caused by exposure to rubella. The court accepted that had the mother known of the real risk to the foetus she would have undergone an abortion. The parents were awarded compensation for the cost to them of raising a severely disabled child whom they would have preferred not to have been born. In awarding compensation to parents in such circumstances the courts are in effect upholding the legitimacy of abortion on grounds of foetal abnormality. Yet if compensation were refused the law would be seen to permit negligent professional conduct to go undeterred.

In *Salih* it was the parents who sued for the wrongful birth of a child. Could the child have sued contending that it would be better for him never to have been born? Such a claim is often called a claim for wrongful life. The Court of Appeal ruled in *McKay* v. *Essex AHA* (1982) that such claims will not be allowed in England. Mary McKay was born in 1970. She suffered from severe abnormalities related to exposure to rubella in the womb. Like Mrs Salih, Mrs McKay had been negligently told that there was no risk that her foetus was endangered by that disease. On Mary's behalf her parents sought compensation from the health authority and their GP arguing that their negligence caused Mary to be born to what would be a life of disability and suffering. The Court of Appeal rejected Mary's claim on the following grounds:

1. It was not possible to assess the proper measure of compensation to represent the difference between never being born at all and being born disabled.
2. If Mary's claim was allowed the law would be imposing a duty to abort.
3. To impose a duty to abort would infringe principles of sanctity of life and devalue disabled members of society generally.

But are those grounds consistent and logical? If parents can sue because professional negligence deprives them of the opportunity to terminate a pregnancy where the foetus is likely to be severely disabled, has the law not already imposed a duty to abort? What is clear is that the judges in *McKay* were considerably disturbed by the moral debate on the status of the foetus and consequently the legitimacy of abortion.

The law governing abortion

As can be seen, allowing a child when born alive to recover compensation for prenatal injuries from some third party who deprived his or her parent of the capacity to have a whole and healthy child does not really raise any substantial ethical problems. If your careless treatment of the mother damages the foetus too, few would disagree that 'both your patients' should receive the protection of the law. Moral debate is provoked when the essence of the argument becomes, as in wrongful life and wrongful birth claims, that you should never have allowed that child to be born at all. Immediately you are at the heart of the debate on the legitimacy of abortion.

The law governing abortion is rather more complicated than discussion in the media sometimes suggests. Section 58 of the Offences against the Person Act 1861 makes it a criminal offence (punishable by life imprisonment) unlawfully to do any act with intent to procure a miscarriage. The woman herself is only guilty of an offence if it can be shown that she actually was pregnant. Anyone else commits a crime if he or she does anything designed to induce an abortion regardless of whether the woman in question in fact was ever pregnant or not. The Abortion Act 1967 did not repeal the 1861 Act which made abortion illegal. It simply set out grounds on which termination of pregnancy (induced abortion) would be lawful. If the abortion is carried out within the provisions of the 1967 Act you have a defence to a charge of criminal abortion. In relation to the upper time limit for lawful abortions the 1967 Act has recently been amended by section 37 of the Human Fertilisation and Embryology Act 1990.

There are now in effect five grounds on which abortion is lawful. The pregnancy must be terminated by a registered medical practitioner after two registered medical practitioners have certified in good faith the opinion that either:

1. The pregnancy is less than twenty-four weeks advanced and the continuation of the pregnancy involves a risk of injury to the physical or mental health of the woman, or of her existing children, greater than if the pregnancy were terminated.
2. At any stage in the pregnancy the continuation of the pregnancy threatens the life of the mother.
3. At any stage in the pregnancy termination of the pregnancy is necessary to prevent grave permanent injury to the physical or mental health of the mother.
4. At any stage in the pregnancy there is a substantial risk that if the child is born it would suffer from such physical or mental abnormalities as to be seriously handicapped.
5. Exceptionally, a single doctor can act unilaterally where abortion is the only means of averting an immediate risk to the life of, or of grave permanent injury to the health of, the pregnant woman.

The vast majority of abortions carried out are performed on the first ground provided for in the amended 1967 Act. The pregnancy is of less than twenty-four weeks' gestation and doctors judge that the risk of continuing the pregnancy and childbirth itself is greater than the risk entailed in induced abortion. English law does not then sanction abortion on demand. It appears to value the foetus, allowing destruction only if the mother's interest in her own health is threatened. Reality is rather different. Many obstetricians now take the liberal view that abortion ought to be the woman's choice. There are statistics on maternal mortality and morbidity which suggest that termination in the first trimester of pregnancy is always safer than continuing the pregnancy to term. Hence some obstetricians argue that abortion in that first twelve weeks of pregnancy is always justifiable under the 1967 Act. By no means all obstetricians adhere to this view. The availability of early abortion can thus vary dramatically depending on whereabouts in the country you live. If you live in an area where obstetricians take a liberal view of abortion, abortion is effectively available on request. In one or two parts of England abortion, save for grave risks to health, may be entirely unobtainable on the NHS.

Note that whatever the justification for allowing the abortion, the termination of the pregnancy must be carried out by a medical practitioner. In 1967, when the Act was passed, all abortions in effect required surgical intervention. Some years later prostaglandin inductions were introduced for later abortions. A doctor inserts a catheter into the woman's womb. Then nursing staff attach the catheter to a pump feeding the hormone prostaglandin into the uterus and induce premature labour. Nurses also fix up a drip into the arm to stimulate contractions. Obviously the foetus is intended to be 'born dead'. The nurse carries out most of the steps required to ensure this end and plays a leading role in terminating the pregnancy. The Royal College of Nursing became concerned that nurses might be breaking the law as under the 1967 Act only doctors could lawfully terminate a pregnancy and they sought an advisory opinion from the courts. Ultimately the Law Lords ruled that the purpose of the Act was to allow for safe, hygienic abortion where that procedure was judged justifiable in the mother's interests or to prevent foetal impairment. Not every physical act necessary to end the pregnancy need be performed by a doctor, but a doctor must undertake overall responsibility for the termination and a nurse acting under his instructions in conformity with standard practice is not in breach of the law (*Royal College of Nursing* v. *DHSS* (1981)).

Nurses may well find participation in abortion distressing whatever their philosophical position on the mother's right to choose to end her pregnancy. As we noted earlier a nurse has a right to refuse to participate in any procedure designed to end the pregnancy, a right enshrined in section 4 of the 1967 Act. However, that right of conscientious objection is legally as well as professionally limited to acts directly relevant to destroying the embryo. A receptionist who refused to type abortion referral letters was found to be outside the protection of section 4 and was held to have been lawfully dismissed for her 'disobedience' (*Janaway* v. *Salford AHA* (1988)). The recent amendment of the 1967 Act in relation to time limits for lawful abortion may cause concern to some nurses who have no fundamental objection to first trimester abortions. For abortion on grounds of foetal impairment can now be carried out at any stage in pregnancy. A child who could be born alive can be destroyed if doctors judge the risk of severe disability is sufficiently great.

The legal regulation of childbirth

Birth remains in the law the crucial watershed. Once the child is delivered, any act designed to kill the newborn infant constitutes murder. There is as such no general crime of infanticide. All the law provides for is that a mother who kills her child of less than a year while her mind is disturbed by childbirth or lactation may escape conviction for murder and be convicted of the lesser offence of infanticide. The nurse who kills or allows an infant to die by neglect is as much guilty of homicide as she would be were her patient an adult. The law's interest in the birth of healthy children is witnessed both by the provision made for compensation for prenatal injury and the limitations still placed on abortion. That interest in the welfare of the child increases as birth approaches. How far does protection of the interests of the child conflict with the interests of the mother and her right to autonomy?

First, Parliament has directly restricted the labouring woman's choice of care. It is a criminal offence under section 17 of the Nurses, Midwives and Health Visitors Act 1979 for any person other than a registered midwife or medical practitioner to attend a woman in childbirth, save in an emergency. Women have a stark choice. Give birth alone or accept professional help. The imposition of this requirement was originally designed to enhance the status of professional midwives and outlaw unhygienic 'handywomen'. But do not think that the rule today is a mere formality. In 1982 a husband was fined £100 for complying with his wife's wishes that he assist her in childbirth.

If mothers in effect must accept professional help what happens if the mother refuses professional advice? The obstetrician may advise that a Caesarean section is necessary in the interests of the baby and the mother may disagree. In the USA courts have enforced surgery and other interventions on unwilling mothers. The courts in effect treated the about-to-be-born as they would a born child and gave precedence to the child's welfare over maternal autonomy. A distressing case in which a woman dying of cancer was forced to undergo Caesarean surgery in a futile attempt to save the foetus has slowed down the rate of judicial intervention across the Atlantic. The position in England is unclear. The question first came before the English courts in the case of *Re F (in utero)* (1988). F had a history of mental disturbance, her first child was already in care and had been given up for adoption. Despite her background psychiatrists found that she was not so disturbed as to warrant detention under the Mental Health Act 1983. She had told the obstetrician that her baby was a reincarnated spirit and refused to go into hospital because she did not trust the doctors or nurses. She then disappeared. The local authority sought to trace the mother and confine her to hospital. They asked the Court of Appeal to make the foetus a ward of court and compel its mother to act in its interests. Their Lordships refused and held that they had no jurisdiction to ward a child before its birth. The four main reasons for this decision were as follows:

1. The foetus has no independent legal rights of its own until it has been born and has an existence separate from its mother.

2. To give the foetus such an enforceable right would be hard to justify in connection with the law on abortion.
3. Extending the wardship jurisdiction to unborn children would require that the interests of the child were paramount and this would thereby conflict with the existing legal interests of the mother.
4. Finally and most practically, there would be tremendous difficulties in enforcing an order to protect the rights of an unborn child against the mother.

However, in 1992 the President of the Family Division gave a surprising judgment in the case of *Re S* which raised issues of both autonomy and consent and the conflicting rights of mother and foetus. He authorised surgeons and staff to carry out a Caesarean section against the wishes of the mother. It was felt by the court to be in the best interests of the mother and to be necessary to protect the interests of the unborn child. While the American courts have retreated from the trend of coercive treatments on pregnant women this case sets a potentially dangerous example in England. In America it has been highlighted that such cases of coercive treatments were most often performed on women from ethnic minorities and under-privileged members of society. In a number of cases, where the women managed to evade the court officials, the children were born healthy without the 'necessary' intervention. The implications of such forcible interventions are worrying. The decisions of competent patients are being overridden because the patient is pregnant. There is no other situation in which a person is obliged to undergo surgery to save another person's life. S, like a number of the women in the American cases, was not afforded legal or medical representation at court. Finally, there are the practical considerations of enforcing such orders, if made in advance, which were considered in *Re F*. What follows from *Re S* remains to be seen but while abortion is permitted in certain cases without time limit, the legal status of the unborn child and the rights of the pregnant mother are now even less clear.

9

Nursing the sick child

Caring for sick children makes obvious emotional and professional demands on the nurse. The especial vulnerability of the very sick child imposes onerous obligations on both his parents and the professionals who look after him, who must often make decisions on his behalf. Defining the ethical and legal responsibilities of the nurse to her child patients is not always easy. The range of potential ethical and legal dilemmas confronting the nurse is awesome. Should the severely disabled, low birthweight, premature infant be treated at all? Is it right to tell a nine-year-old that he is HIV positive? Can a fourteen-year-old girl be prescribed the Pill without her parents' knowledge? How do you respond when you suspect a child has been abused by a parent? Should a sixteen-year-old anorexic be forced to eat? The diversity of the problems posed by caring for children has, however, two common themes in terms of ethical and legal debate, as follows: firstly, when a child cannot make treatment decisions for himself, must parental decisions on his behalf always be respected? Secondly, at what stage in his development does a child acquire a capacity to make his own decisions? When must he be treated as an autonomous individual? In 1989 the Children Act was enacted to reform the law relating to both the care of children whose parents were separated, and the public protection of children whose parents were unable to care for them themselves. The Act was hailed as a new dawn for respect for children's rights. The media presented the legislation as a comprehensive code governing all aspects of decision-making relating to children. As you will see, in relation to health care, the Children Act does have relevance to the care of child patients but is perhaps not quite as all-pervasive as you might expect.

Neonatal care: ethical considerations

Modern neonatal intensive care offers babies once considered impossible to treat a chance of survival. However, as in all areas of health care which are dependent upon high technological care, there is an ethical dimension to consider. Concern centres around three broad groups of infants, those born at the limits of viability, that is, around twenty-four weeks gestation, those with congenital abnormalities especially involving the brain and spinal cord, and those who are injured either during delivery or as a result of disease in pregnancy.

The usual practice when a baby is born pre-term is to resuscitate and then transfer the baby to a neonatal unit so that the baby may receive intensive care to stabilise his condition. Not all hospitals have neonatal intensive care facilities, so if a pre-term birth is anticipated, the woman may be transferred to a hospital which has such facilities prior to delivery, or alternatively if there is no time to move the mother, then the baby may be transferred immediately after birth. A baby who needs to be transferred in this way is at a disadvantage, and clearly there are inequalities in the neonatal care facilities throughout the country as intensive care facilities tend to be situated in hospitals in large towns and cities. Many babies do respond to treatment and even after prolonged periods spent in a neonatal care unit are able to live normal lives. For others, the response to the treatment is less successful and they go on to develop further complications with iatrogenic causes. A minority overall respond poorly to treatment and then a decision needs to be made whether treatment should be discontinued.

If a baby is not responding to treatment, it may be the considered medical and nursing opinion that further treatment is futile, that it should be stopped and the baby allowed to die. Neonatal paediatricians such as Campbell, Duff and Whitelaw have detailed their methods for dealing with situations of this sort in their own units and have as a consequence opened up the debate in a more public arena. This is a controversial subject which is further complicated by the role that the parents play in the decision-making process. Many of the arguments are similar to those put forward when caring for adults who are terminally ill or reaching the end of their life, but the issue is often seen as being more emotive when babies are concerned. Another sort of case too must be discussed in relation to very sick babies. It may be that on diagnosis of a particular disability a decision is taken not to treat the baby at all. An infant is born with spina bifida and parents and doctors decide not to operate. Or perhaps a baby with Downs' syndrome also suffers from a duodenal atresia and the parents reject the necessary life-saving surgery. In an extreme case a decision might be made not to feed the baby. One case in particular received considerable attention because the paediatrician was charged with murder as a consequence of his actions.

The Leonard Arthur case

On 28 June 1980 in Derby, John Pearson was born. He was diagnosed as having Down's syndrome shortly after delivery and examined by Dr Leonard

Arthur, a consultant paediatrician, the same day. Following his examination of the baby and discussions with the parents, Dr Arthur recorded in the baby's notes that the parents did not wish the baby to survive, that the baby was to be given nursing care only and he prescribed 5mg of DF118 to be given when required at the discretion of the nurse in charge but no more than every four hours. DF118 is a strong analgesic drug not usually prescribed for children and Down's syndrome is not a painful condition so analgesic drugs should not have been required. Although the record of events is vague, it appears that John Pearson was regularly given 'feeds' of water and DF118 until he died on 1 July 1980. A member of the hospital staff reported the case to Life, a pro-life organisation who subsequently reported the case to the police and Dr Arthur was charged with murder.

Initially it was thought that John Pearson did not have any of the life-threatening abnormalities sometimes associated with Down's syndrome, but pathologists giving evidence in Dr Arthur's defence proved conclusively that the baby in fact had abnormalities of the heart, lung and brain which may have contributed to the his death. As a result, halfway through the trial the charge was changed from murder to attempted murder. The jury ultimately found Dr Arthur not guilty (R v. Arthur (1981)).

This case raised several ethical issues. First of all, a decision clearly had been made that John Pearson should not live and measures were taken to ensure that he did not do so. Some would argue that acting in this way has no moral distinction from killing the baby immediately, say, by giving him a lethal injection. If health professionals think that one method is acceptable then perhaps the other should be also. This distinction between killing and letting die will be fully discussed in Chapter Twelve. Cases of this sort are challenging for the nurses concerned with the care of the baby as after a decision has been made to allow a baby to die, it is the responsibility of the nurses involved to care for the baby until he does die. And they must interpret what constitutes nursing care only.

The acquittal of Dr Arthur leaves another ethical dilemma unresolved. Dr Arthur accepted the baby's parents' decision to reject treatment of their child simply because he had Down's syndrome. Remember that at the time that it was decided to provide nursing care only, both Dr Arthur and the parents were unaware of his additional disabilities. Accepting the parental judgment implies either that parents have a general power of life or death over their children or that society recognises that some lives are not worth saving and that disabled infants are of less value than their unimpaired siblings. The personhood argument discussed in relation to abortion is relevant again here. Philosophers such as Harris and Singer might argue that if the newborn lacks the capacities on which personhood depends, he has no independent moral rights of his own. His parents are entitled to let or help him die. After all, had his disability been discovered at any time prior to birth he could have been lawfully aborted. Such arguments will be entirely unacceptable to those holding traditional views on the sanctity of human life.

Discontinuing treatment

A more common scenario than the Arthur case is that emergency treatment is administered at birth, but later if the baby makes no progress, a decision may be made to discontinue the treatment. Suppose that a baby born at twenty-four weeks gestation has been admitted to a neonatal intensive care unit. The baby has been mechanically ventilated for two weeks and has made little or no progress during this time. Investigations show that there are signs of severe neurological damage and that the baby, even if he survives, will be severely physically and mentally disabled. It may be argued that treatment should be discontinued in the interests of the baby; it cannot be to the child's advantage to be kept alive only to lead a life restricted by severe physical and mental disability. This is a consequentialist argument and may be extended to include consideration of the interests of the parents, other members of the family and society in general.

One of the problems of arguing in this way is that it is difficult to assess what quality of life this baby may be said to have. For someone who does not have any form of physical or mental disability, the prospect would probably seem bleak. We would naturally think of the things in our life we would be unable to continue doing, but we are only able to do this because we have had the experience of living a life unhampered by disability and have the perception to know the difference. A person with a mental disability who does not have that perception would be unable to make this comparison and as a consequence may not think he has a poor quality of life. Clearly this will depend upon the family that the baby is born into, but if a family is prepared to accept such a child despite any difficulties that may arise, then in some respects the child may be considered as having a good quality of life.

The consequentialist is not necessarily committed to saying that treatment should be discontinued in this case, as consideration may also be given to the interests of society as a whole. It may be suggested that by arguing that treatment should be discontinued, then what is really being said is that the life of a disabled person is not worth living and this could affect the status of existing disabled people in society. If babies with disabilities are not treated, this may change people's attitudes to existing disabled people so that they are discriminated against. The consequentialist may thus contend that by discontinuing treatment of babies wih abnormalities you potentially cause harm to existing disabled people, and therefore treatment should not be discontinued.

The disabled newborn

We have already seen that it is no longer the uniform practice to treat every infant born alive regardless of degree of abnormality, and that when treatment of very sick newborns is initiated it may be discontinued if doctors and parents judge that the baby's prospects of survival and/or a decent quality of life are slim. Leonard Arthur was acquitted of the attempted murder of John Pearson, but that decision tells us little of what the law requires in such a case. One point must be made absolutely clear. Once the baby is born, the law regards her or him as having a legal personality equivalent to yours or ours. Any deliberate act designed to hasten the death of the infant constitutes murder. And if a person responsible for an infant deliberately withholds care treatment from that infant with the intention that the baby should die, that too constitutes murder just as much as if she put a pillow over the child's face. When a father and his mistress in effect starved his child to death both were convicted of murder (*R* v. *Gibbins and Proctor* (1918). Much more recently parents who failed to obtain appropriate treatment for their diabetic daughter were convicted of manslaughter when the child died. However, just as with an adult, the duty to provide appropriate care for a patient does not demand that life be prolonged at all costs and in all circumstances. The professional and the parental duty is to provide appropriate care in the best interests of the infant. When does the law recognise that allowing a severely damaged infant to die is truly in the child's best interests?

The case law concerning babies with a disability

A much more instructive legal judgment than the trial of Dr Arthur can be found in the judgment of the Court of Appeal in *Re B* (1981). Like John Pearson, baby Alexandra was also born in 1981 with Down's syndrome. She additionally suffered from an intestinal obstruction which prevented normal digestion. On the 2 per cent of children born with this defect, the necessary operation is normally performed within a few hours of birth. It carries very little risk and is usually successful. However, in the light of her disability, Alexandra's parents decided that she should not have the operation and should be allowed to die a natural death. Members of the health care team looking after Alexandra differed as to how the problem should be approached. The surgeon refused to operate without the parents' consent but other practitioners on the unit disagreed. Ultimately the dispute on Alexandra's fate was referred to the courts. The Court of Appeal ordered that the operation should go ahead on the basis that such routine treatment should never be withheld unless evidence could be adduced to the effect that the child's life would be 'demonstrably awful'. Lord Justice Templeman said:

It is a decision which of course must be made in the light of evidence and views expressed by the parents and the doctors, but at the end of the day it devolves on this court in this particular instance to decide whether the life of this child is demonstrably going to be so awful that in effect the child must be condemned to die, or whether the life of this child is still so imponderable that it would be wrong for her to be condemned to die. There may be cases, I know not, of severe proved damage where the future is so certain and where the life of the child is so bound to be full of pain and suffering that the court might be driven to a different conclusion, but in the present case the choice which lies before the court is this: whether to allow an operation to take place which may result in the child living for twenty or thirty years as a mongoloid or whether (and I think this brutally must be the result) to terminate the life of a mongoloid child because she also has an intestinal complaint. Faced with that choice I have no doubt that it is the duty of this court to decide that the child must live. (p. 929)

Yet in that same year Dr Arthur had been acquitted of attempted murder in leaving another Down's syndrome baby to die. And in a third case in 1981 the Government refused to prosecute doctors who had decided not to operate on an infant with severe spina bifida. Further clarification of the law had to await a second trio of cases between 1989 and 1992.

In *Re C* in 1989, C was born with severe hydrocephalus and brain deformities for which there was no hope of successful treatment. For some months C lived in the paediatric unit of the hospital but it was becoming more difficult to feed her. It became apparent that she was blind and probably deaf; her responses to anything were poor and natural feeding was becoming impossible. The question was whether the nursing and medical staff were obliged to keep her alive by artificial, intravenous feeding and whether they must treat any infection that she was likely to succumb to. The medical evidence indicated that C would die within a few months whatever treatment was given to her. But C's social worker insisted that the staff must do whatever they would do for a 'normal' baby. This became the fundamental issue; whether a baby with severe disabilities should be treated in the same way as any other child. The Court of Appeal took the view that as C was in the process of dying the decision as to her treatment should be left with those who had her in their care. Where death was simply being prolonged the staff could lawfully withhold treatment. Their duty was to do whatever was necessary to minimise C's suffering.

The following year saw the appeal court again considering the fate of a severely disabled infant *Re J* (1990). J was born three months prematurely and suffered severe and permanent brain damage. It was likely that he would develop serious spastic quadriplegia. He was largely blind and deaf but did respond to his carers and his projected lifespan might well continue into his teens. On two occasions he had stopped breathing and had to be mechanically ventilated. The question put to the court was whether if he stopped breathing again he must be resuscitated. Both J's parents and his health carers felt that he should not be, but they feared prosecution if they simply went ahead and let J die. The crucial distinction between C and J is, of course, that J was not imminently dying regardless of what might be done for him.

The Court of Appeal ruled that there was no obligation to ventilate J. A balancing exercise must be performed when considering the best interests of the infant. The opinions of family and medical staff must be weighed. The child's perspective on his future life must be assessed to determine whether, to use Lord Justice Templeman's words from *Re B*, his life will be so 'demonstrably awful' that death is preferable to life. Lord Donaldson put it this way: '. . . in the end there will be cases in which the answer must be that it is not in the interests of the child to subject it to treatment which will cause increased suffering and produce no commensurate benefit, giving the fullest possible weight to the child's, and mankind's desire to survive' (p. 938).

So in both *Re C* and *Re J* the law sanctioned judgments by those caring for the sick infant that it was not in her or his interests to have life prolonged by heroic therapy or artificial feeding. But the painful dilemma of whether to continue to treat a very damaged infant is made even worse if those responsible for the child disagree as they did in the second case also entitled *Re J* in 1992. One month after he was born in January 1991, J sustained serious head injuries which resulted in profound mental and physical disability. The consensus of medical opinion was that he would be unlikely to develop much beyond his present state and had an uncertain life expectancy. He suffered intermittent convulsive attacks which required resuscitative treatment. The consultant paediatrician, with whom the health authority and other practitioners concurred, felt that it was medically inappropriate to use mechanical ventilation procedures in any future attack. His mother vehemently disagreed. She wanted the court to order the doctors to carry out the treatment including ventilating her son if that was necessary to prolong his life.

The Court of Appeal refused to order doctors to ventilate J. Lord Donaldson stated, 'the law is clear. The question whether artificial ventilation should or should not be applied is . . . an entirely medical one with which the courts will not interfere' (p. 514). He went on to say:

> The fundamental issue in this appeal is whether the court in the exercise of its inherent power to protect the interests of minors should ever require a medical practitioner or health authority acting by a medical practitioner to adopt a course of treatment which in the bona fide clinical judgment of the practitioner concerned is contra-indicated as not being in the best interests of the patient. I have to say that I cannot at present conceive of any circumstances

in which this would be other than an abuse of power as directly or indirectly requiring the practitioner to act contrary to the fundamental duty which he owes to his patient. This, subject to obtaining any necessary consent, is to treat the patient in accordance with his own best clinical judgment, notwithstanding that other practitioners who are called upon to treat the patient may have formed a quite different judgment or that the court, acting on expert evidence, may disagree with him. (p. 516)

It is nigh on impossible to establish hard and fast rules from the case law relating to infants with severe disabilities. Each case turns largely on its own facts – what course of action is in the best interests of that particular baby? Clearly parents cannot demand that doctors treat a child when the medical prognosis is that treatment is futile. Equally clearly parents cannot refuse treatment on their own subjective assessment of their baby's interests. The practical advice to health care staff must be that faced with a dilemma over whether to treat or to continue to treat a sick newborn or small infant, you should seek the assistance of the courts. This can be done in several ways, either by invoking section 100 of the Children Act 1989 and the inherent jurisdiction of the courts to protect minors or by way of seeking a specific issue order under that same Act. The rather complex procedural steps involved are beyond our remit but be assured whatever procedure is followed, the courts in cases involving sick children can act swiftly, flexibly and with compassion. Once a case is referred to the court, the judge's role is to adjudicate on the infant's best interest. Note two aspects of the judicial exercise. First, the English courts operate a presumption in favour of life. Lord Justice Taylor said in *Re J* (1990): 'the court's high respect for the sanctity of human life imposes a strong presumption in favour of taking all steps capable of preserving it, save in exceptional circumstances' (p. 943).

Second, the courts pay perhaps undue deference to medical opinion. Treatment which responsible medical opinion considers not to be beneficial to the child is unlikely to be sanctioned regardless of the contrary opinion of the parents. It sometimes seems doctors rather than parents are treated as primarily responsible for the child patient. Lord Donaldson in *Re J* (1990) put it this way.

The doctors owe the child a duty to care for it in accordance with good medical practice recognised as appropriate by a competent body of professional opinion ... This duty is, however, subject to the qualification that, if time permits, they must obtain the consent of the parents before undertaking serious invasive treatment. The parents owe the child a duty to give or to withhold consent in the best interests of the child and without regard to their own interests. The court when exercising the *parens patriae* jurisdiction takes over the rights and duties of the parents, although this is not to say that the parents will be excluded from the decision-making process. Nevertheless the decision whether to give or to withhold consent is that of the court alone.

What is a child?

When caring for any child, health professionals face difficulties in the areas of confidentiality and respect for autonomy, particularly when consent is required for an invasive procedure, for surgery or for the child to participate in research. Although in normal circumstances, parents would be involved in any decisions regarding their child, it is unrealistic to expect that the parents will always be clear about what actions will be in the best interests of their child. Not all that long ago children were viewed as the property of their parents, but the current emphasis is now on society's responsibility for the protection of children and their interests.

Because of the nature of her role, the nurse may find herself the child's confidant or advocate and may be faced with ethical dilemmas as a consequence of this role. She may find herself in conflict with the child's parents while attempting to safeguard the interests of the child. In many respects, one fundamental problem that lies beneath all of these issues centres on what our definition of a child is.

In English law you do not become an adult, or come of age, until you are eighteen. Everyone under eighteen is classified as a minor and her or his capacity is in certain respects limited by the law for her or his own protection. However, that does not mean that every person under eighteen is deprived of the right and ability to take any decisions for herself or himself. We are not faced with the absurd scenario that only the parents of a boy of seventeen and a half can decide if he may have his broken arm set. The law accords with common sense in recognising that maturity is an evolutionary process and, as we shall see, presumes a capacity to make decisions about health care at sixteen while still accepting that in a number of instances children younger than sixteen are capable of deciding certain matters for themselves. We look at the intricacies of the legal rules later. The first question we need to ask is: when should we begin to accord an older child the respect due to an autonomous being? Children grow up at different speeds. Arbitrary age limits on autonomy are unhelpful, and we need to concentrate on the individual child in our care. The difficulty is deciding exactly when a child is mature enough to understand and make decisions about her or his own life. This will vary from child to child and will for example depend on the child's ability to understand, the relationship with parents and the child's previous experiences. For example, a child with cancer who has had numerous admissions to hospital, a variety of treatments and surgery, may demonstrate a far greater level of understanding and maturity than a child who has never been seriously ill or admitted to hospital. In most situations, health professionals will need to consider each child separately in the light of her or his own particular circumstances, but there is, as a result of this, potential for conflict between health professionals, the child and the child's parents or guardians.

Children and consent

Obviously there are many situations when caring for sick children when consent will need to be obtained either from a child or from the child's parents. In the majority of cases this will be straightforward but in some circumstances there may be conflict which will raise ethical questions for health professionals involved in caring for the child. A recent case which received media attention illustrates the potential for such conflict. A four-year-old child diagnosed as having a brain tumour was prescribed a course of radiotherapy treatment. There was only a 30 per cent chance that this treatment would cure the child and his mother decided that she did not wish her son to be subjected to this treatment. The reasons she gave were the poor chance of the treatment being successful and the fact that the child had previously undergone chemotherapy treatment which in itself had made the child even more ill. The doctors caring for the child considered taking court action so that the child could be treated irrespective of his mother's wishes even though his mother stated that the child himself had repeatedly asked to be allowed to die because of the pain he was suffering.

The question which needs to be answered in this case is who is acting in the child's best interests? Are the doctors, who want to cure the child and therefore will administer any treatment that offers some chance of a cure? Or is it the mother, who feels that the child has experienced enough suffering and should not be subjected to any further treatment that will cause more suffering and offers only a limited chance of curing her son? The attitude of the doctors is perhaps understandable as they obviously feel that while there is some form of treatment available which will offer the chance of a cure then it should be taken. So much so, they were prepared to take the necessary legal steps to override his mother's decision, although it may be argued that in acting in this way they stressed only the physical interests of the child. On the other hand, his mother, while still concerned about the physical interests of her son, also placed emphasis on protecting his psychological and emotional interests.

Although such a case could be settled in a court of law and a practical solution found for this dilemma, a judge would not necessarily give a satisfactory moral answer. If the court ruled in favour of the doctor's decision, then the autonomous decision made by the child's mother would be overridden and this would have implications for other situations when parents need to make decisions on behalf of their children. Alternatively, if the court ruled in favour of the mother, then the child would die whereas with the treatment he might have some chance of being cured.

It would be convenient for health care professionals if we could agree on a precise age when a child is capable of making a truly autonomous decision for himself. Alas, that is not possible. Autonomy does not appear overnight. The capacity to act autonomously evolves as the child grows up and is, as we have seen, very much influenced by the child's individual understanding and experience. The lawyer must be concerned with the one act of giving consent. Has treatment been lawfully authorised by parent or child? Ethically the process of obtaining consent is much more crucial. Have the professionals provided the degree and quality of information about the proposed treatment to enable parents and the child to decide what to do next? Does that individual child have a sufficient understanding of that information for her or his opinion on accepting or rejecting treatment to carry weight? Is the child mature enough to decide what constitute her or his own best interests? Compromise and negotiation about what does constitute those interests must always be preferable to confrontation.

The mother in the above example rejected further treatment of her son because she believed the pain and trauma entailed in that treatment outweighed the prospect of recovery. The potential conflict between professionals and parents is exacerbated if parents reject treatment where the prospects of recovery are good and do so, not because they judge that the treatment will cause tangible harm to their child, but on the basis of religious belief. The classic example is parents refusing blood transfusions in conformity with their faith as Jehovah's Witnesses. Autonomy entitles the parents to have any judgment that they themselves should not receive blood respected. But can that judgment be enforced upon a child who has not yet independently decided to follow her or his parents' faith and not yet judged death preferable to violation of the faith? We would suggest not and that the professionals' responsibility in such a case is to ensure that the child lives by resorting to legal action if necessary. Two reservations should, however, be expressed. First, the parents' beliefs are entitled to respect. Unnecessary, heavy-handed intervention will damage the family and damage the child. Second, of course, the older child moving towards autonomy may support her or his parents' judgment. Would you consider it right to coerce an intelligent fifteen-year-old into receiving blood? If your answer is yes, why is this so if you would (albeit reluctantly) accept the decision of her twenty-five-year-old brother?

Children and confidentiality

Parents in their desire to protect their child may attempt to withhold information about the child's illness from the child and request that health professionals respect this confidentiality. This can cause two main difficulties. Firstly, the child may question her or his carers about the nature of the illness so that the nurse or any other health professional has difficulty in being honest with the child. Secondly, the nurse may believe that the parents are misguided and that not only does the child have a right to know the facts but it is necessary that he or she does so. Suppose that Steven, a sixteen-year-old man with haemophilia, has in the past contracted HIV as the result of a contaminated blood transfusion. His parents do not want their son to be made aware of this and ask that the staff ensure that he is not given this information. During a period of hospital admission for treatment, Steven confides in the nurse that he has recently formed a relationship with a young woman and although this has not yet developed into a sexual relationship, they have discussed this possibility. The nurse is faced with a dilemma because she wants to respect the wishes of the parents, but clearly feels that it is vital that Steven is given information about his HIV status before embarking on any sexual relationship. The nurse could argue that in her role as the patient's advocate, her primary responsibilities are to patients and clients, and decide to go against the parents' wishes and inform Steven herself. After all, it is Steven, and not his parents, who is her patient.

Children and the law

The fundamental questions posed by the law in relation to the care of sick children are straightforward. While a child is too young to take any sort of decision for herself or himself, who is entitled to act on her or his behalf? At what stage in development does the child acquire the legal capacity to act for herself or himself? When does the law intervene to protect the child either against decisions made for her or him by parents or professionals, or, in the case of older children, against their own decisions?

From infancy to childhood

The principles established in the case law relating to severely disabled babies are theoretically applicable to any non-autonomous child. Neither C nor J (1990) were strictly speaking neonates as both were sixteen weeks old. Various proposals have been made to legislate specifically for the non-treatment of impaired neonates but none have come to fruition. So if a two-year-old is devastatingly injured in a road accident, or a six-year-old develops a brain tumour, that same balancing exercise to determine if his life will be 'demonstrably awful' must be applied to him as to his infant sister. Where treatment is indisputably in his best interests it can be enforced on him. It is not an assault to inoculate a protesting child, nor to lift his screaming sister into the dentist's chair.

But as the child grows older, we have seen that he or she grows towards autonomy and ethicists argue that his or her own decisions must be respected. We might agree that the protesting four-year-old should be vaccinated for his own good, but should his fourteen-year-old sister be forced to have an abortion? Or, if she wants an abortion, is the consent of her parents required in addition to her own?

Victoria Gillick and the Family Law Reform Act 1969

The Family Law Reform Act 1969 lowered the general age of majority from twenty-one to eighteen. Section 8 of the Act also provides for a 'medical age of majority' at sixteen. The Act states:

1. The consent of a minor who has attained the age of sixteen years to any surgical, medical or dental treatment which, in the absence of consent, would constitute a trespass to his person shall be as effective as it would be if he were of full age: and where a minor has by virtue of this section given an effective consent it shall not be necessary to obtain any consent for it from his parent or guardian.
2. In this section 'surgical, medical or dental treatment' includes any procedure undertaken for the purposes of diagnosis, and this section applies to any procedure (including, in particular, the administration of an anaesthetic) which is ancillary to any treatment as it applies to that treatment.
3. Nothing in this section shall be construed as making ineffective any consent which would have been effective if this section had not been enacted.

What this rather convoluted provision certainly means is this – once someone is sixteen if he or she gives consent to treatment no additional consent is needed from the teenager's parents. If a sixteen-year-old girl seeks contraceptive advice or an abortion, or a seventeen-year-old youth authorises surgery, it is entirely lawful to act on their respective judgments alone. But what of the patient under sixteen? Does the law treat autonomy as acquired on, and not before, the sixteenth birthday? Most lawyers interpreted section 8 of the Family Law Reform Act to mean that health care professionals could treat anyone over sixteen as competent to consent to treatment, but in the case of a child under sixteen they must assess whether that individual child was capable of deciding for herself or himself on the treatment in issue. Victoria Gillick challenged that assumption, arguing that until a child reached sixteen only her parents could give a valid consent to treatment.

The Gillick case – the facts

The highly publicised *Gillick* litigation was generated by a circular issued by the DHSS in 1974. In trying to combat the growing numbers of under-age pregnancies and abortions, the circular advised that it was lawful to treat and prescribe contraceptives for girls under sixteen without contacting the parents if the girl understood what was entailed and the doctor judged that providing her with contraceptive treatment was in the girl's best interests. The 1980 version of the circular urged doctors to make every effort to involve parents but if a girl was adamant that her parents should not know, the doctor should respect the relationship of confidentiality between doctor and child patient, and parents should not be told.

Mrs Gillick was, at the time, the mother of four daughters under sixteen. She sought to argue that providing contraception to a girl under sixteen was illegal. She relied on two rather different arguments. First, she contended that as sexual intercourse with a girl under sixteen constitutes a criminal offence, a doctor providing such a girl with contraceptive treatment or advice was aiding and abetting the commission of a crime. Second, she maintained that while a child was under sixteen any medical treatment of the child constituted a battery unless authorised by a parent or the courts. Attempts to obtain assurances from her local health authority that none of her own daughters would be given contraception without her consent failed and so she resorted to legal action seeking declarations that it would be unlawful to give any of her daughters under sixteen contraceptive or abortion advice or treatment without her prior knowledge and consent.

The House of Lords ultimately ruled by a majority that providing contraception to girls under sixteen did not amount to assisting her partner to have unlawful sexual intercourse with her. Simply providing contraception to a girl who has already embarked, or is determined to embark on, a sexual relationship in order to protect her against pregnancy is not facilitating or encouraging the unlawful act. The doctor does no more than offer 'a palliative against the consequences of crime'. Health professionals must tread carefully though when providing contraception to under-age girls. They must not in any sense encourage premature sexual relations. Lord Fraser offered the following guidance to the health care professional confronted by a young person seeking contraceptive advice or treatment. He must satisfy himself:

> (1) that the girl . . . will understand his advice; (2) that he cannot persuade her to inform her parents . . . ; (3) that she is very likely to begin or continue having sexual intercourse with or without contraceptive treatment; (4) that unless she receives contraceptive advice or treatment her physical or mental health or both are likely to suffer; (5) that her best interests require him to give her contraceptive advice or treatment or both without the parental consent. (p. 413)

Mrs Gillick lost too on her second argument that any treatment of a child under sixteen was unlawful in the absence of parental consent. The Law Lords held that once a child 'achieves a sufficient understanding and intelligence to enable him or her to understand fully what is proposed' the child can give a valid consent to treatment. In other words, once the child is capable of making an autonomous judgment, she can authorise treatment for herself. Parental rights to authorise treatment of their younger children derive from parental responsibilities to ensure their children receive adequate health care when needed. Those rights dwindle as the child grows up and becomes able to take responsibility for herself. As Lord Scarman put it: 'the parental right yields to the child's right to make his own decisions when he reaches a sufficient understanding and intelligence to be capable of making up his own mind on the matter requiring decision'.

The *Gillick* case echoes the ethical debate in refusing to set a precise age for capacity to consent to treatment. Each child must be assessed individually in the light of the particular treatment proposed. An intelligent fourteen-year-old may well be capable of consenting to treatment to regulate heavy periods, but not to sterilisation to avert the risk that she will give birth to a haemophiliac son. Before acting on the consent of any child alone a health care professional must be very sure that that child truly understands what she is agreeing to. He must be able to demonstrate that the child is '*Gillick* competent'.

Confidentiality and children under sixteen

A girl under sixteen seeking contraceptive advice is often going to be as much concerned about her parents hearing of her request as whether she has the capacity to give a valid consent to treatment. However, courts in *Gillick* paid little attention to the issue of confidentiality. The House of Lords held that in certain circumstances the doctor was free to treat the girl without parental knowledge. The question remains whether or not a doctor or nurse is obliged to respect and observe the girl's confidentiality. The House of Lords upheld the DHSS guidelines and thereby impliedly endorsed the view that the doctor or nurse owed a duty of confidentiality to the patient under sixteen. None the less the problems relating to bringing an action for breach of confidence have already been discussed in Chapter Five. There it was seen that the duty of confidentiality is generally given more effective support in the UKCC *Code of Professional Conduct* and established professional practice than by the law. Moreover '*Gillick* competence' depends on the health care professional being satisfied that the girl has the understanding and maturity to agree to treatment, to be treated in effect as an adult.

Consent and younger children

In each case involving a sick child the health care worker must assess the maturity of the individual child to establish whether that child is '*Gillick* competent'. There is no set age limit as to when this stage of development is attained. What is the legal position when a nurse decides that the child is too immature to decide for herself? In the simplest scenario, where a child is sick, caring parents may consent to treatment which is for the child's benefit and their consent will authorise the nurse's actions. There can, if such consent is obtained, be no action for battery. Problems arise in the following scenarios. First, when a parent is not available or is uninterested. Second, when a parent expressly refuses consent to treatment.

In the first scenario the nurse may provide whatever treatment is immediately necessary. Such action may be legally justified using the defence of necessity or by implication based on the presumption that the absent parent would agree to similar treatment for the child. Indeed, in the *Gillick* case Lord Scarman said 'Emergency, parental neglect, abandonment of the child or inability to find the parent are examples of exceptional situations justifying the doctor proceeding to treat the child without parental knowledge and consent.' (p. 424).

The second scenario poses greater legal problems. Take for example the case of a Jehovah's Witness refusing to authorise a blood transfusion for a child. We would argue that in such a situation the health care worker may proceed with treatment where it is immediately necessary to save the child's life or health. Parents themselves are under a duty to provide adequate medical care for their children – failure to do so is to commit the offence of wilful neglect (Children and Young Persons Act 1933 s.1(1)). If the child dies the parent may also face a charge of manslaughter. In *R v. Senior* (1899) the courts held that sincerely held religious conviction is no defence where the parent appreciated the seriousness of the child's condition but refused to seek help.

Lord Templeman explained the position this way in *Gillick*:

> Where the patient is an infant, the medical profession accepts that a parent having custody and being responsible for the infant is entitled on behalf of the infant to consent to or reject treatment if the parent considers that the best interests of the infant so require. Where doctor and parent disagree, the court can decide and is not slow to act. I accept that if there is no time to obtain a decision from the court, a doctor may safely carry out treatment in an emergency if the doctor believes the treatment to be vital to the survival or health of the infant and notwithstanding the opposition of a parent or the impossibility of alerting the parent before the treatment is carried out. (p. 432)

However, unilateral action by health professionals should be avoided unless a child's life is in imminent danger. The dispute between parents and professionals as to the child's best interests should be referred to the Family Division of the High Court, and, as Lord Templeman noted, in this sort of case the courts will act swiftly.

Today there are two routes by which a dispute relating to the medical treatment of a child may reach the courts. Either party to the dispute, the parents or the professionals, may make an application for an order under section 8 of the Children Act. This may be either for a 'specific issue order' requiring that certain action be taken. Or it may be for a 'prohibited steps order' prohibiting a particular procedure. Parents have an unfettered right to apply to the court under section 8. The professionals will have to liaise with local social workers and seek leave to apply to the court. Obviously if the core of the dispute is whether or not a child should receive a trans-fusion the professionals will be asking for a 'specific issue order' author-ising the administration of blood. The parents will want a 'prohibited steps order' banning a treatment contrary to their faith. However, although many people originally saw the Children Act as a kind of 'code' of child law laying down detailed rules as to the resolution of disputes involving children, the courts have recently suggested that it may be preferable to avoid an application under section 8 and take a dispute concerning the medical treatment of a child to court by invoking the inherent jurisdiction of the High Court preserved under section 100 of the Act. That way the court has a wide discretion to do what the judge thinks best for the child and the decision will always be left to a very senior judge. You as a nurse should not become too distracted by the niceties of the legal procedures. Leave that to the lawyers! Whichever means is employed to refer the dispute concerning the child to the court, the dispute will be adjudicated in much the same way. The judge will listen to and evaluate the arguments about the needs and interests of the child. Where spiritual and temporal interests conflict, the latter is likely to prevail if the child's life is at stake. In all the English cases relating to the children of Jehovah's Witnesses so far, the court has ordered that the blood transfusion be carried out. How-ever, you must note that the courts today are sensitive to the parents' sincere conviction and the possible psychological effects on the child of flouting the family faith. If alternatives to blood are realistically available, proper consideration must be given to their use.

Children refusing treatment

The older 'Gillick competent' child acquires the capacity to authorise treat-ment for herself or himself. The younger child will generally rely on his parents to act on his behalf, and determine his best interests in relation to medical treatment. Even if the child objects to that treatment, treatment may still lawfully proceed although every care must be taken to avoid the harm which outright coercion, or even use of force, might occasion the child. But what happens when an older 'Gillick competent' child says no to treatment her parents believe that she should undergo? A fifteen-year-old refuses a fixed brace for fear of alienating her boyfriend. An anorexic girl refuses to eat. After Gillick is it the case that once the child has acquired the maturity to understand what is entailed in treatment she is truly autonomous and can refuse as well as consent to treatment? That seemed to follow from Lord Scarman's declaration that the parental right yielded to the child's right to make her or his own decisions. None the less, in two recent judgments, Re R (1991), and Re W (1992), the Court of Appeal has ruled that no one under eighteen has an absolute right to refuse treatment considered to be in his or her best interests.

The disturbed teenager

R was a fifteen-year-old girl who had endured a traumatic and disrupted childhood. Her psychiatric problems were such that she was placed in an adolescent psychiatric unit and was being treated with anti-psychotic drugs. Her mental state fluctuated between apparent rationality and what were described as 'florid episodes'. She decided to refuse to take her medication. Doctors and social workers examined R but concluded that she was not so mentally disturbed that she could be 'sectioned' under the Mental Health Act 1983 and detained for psychiatric treatment. Had she been 'sectioned' section 63 of the Act would have authorised administering her drugs to her without her consent. R was in the care of the local authority so doctors then asked the local authority to agree that R should be compelled to stay on medication. The local authority referred R's sad dilemma to the courts.

The trial judge listened to the evidence and concluded R was not 'Gillick competent'. She may have been fifteen, but her mental illness deprived her of the insight and understanding necessary to enable a child under sixteen to make treatment decisions for herself. The Court of Appeal agreed. R had not achieved 'Gillick competence' and therefore the court, or whoever had parental responsibility for R, could authorise whatever treatment was in R's best interests. The judgment has been criticised for the way all the judges assessed 'Gillick competence', but a much more important issue was raised in the judgment of the President of the Court of Appeal, Lord Donaldson. He maintained that even if R were 'Gillick competent' she could not veto treatment which others responsible for her believed to be in her interests. He argued that when an older child becomes 'Gillick competent' she acquires the ability to authorise treatment for herself, but her parents' power to authorise treatment on her behalf does not lapse. For medical treatment to be lawful, a valid consent must be obtained. Where the patient is a 'Gillick competent' child that consent may be obtained from the child, or either parent, or the court. He used the analogy of a keyholder opening the door to lawful treatment. While a child is young the parents are the sole keyholders, but the older teenager becomes a keyholder in her own right and any single keyholder can open the door. The effect of Lord Donaldson's argument in *Re R* was that an older child acquired a right to say yes to treatment, but no right to say no.

The anorexic teenager

W was another teenager with a tragic history. She had developed anorexia nervosa after the death of her grandfather. Like R she was in the care of the local authority. When she was sixteen her weight had dropped to six stone and five pounds and she was five foot seven inches tall. Despite earlier co-operation with her doctors she now refused to agree to naso-gastric feeding, and opposed an attempt to move her to a London clinic specialising in eating disorders. An application was made to the court under its inherent jurisdiction and both the trial judge and the Court of Appeal authorised W's removal to the London clinic and declared doctors could, if need be, resort to naso-gastric feeding.

The issue in *Re W* is not whether W was '*Gillick* competent'. She was after all sixteen and, as we have seen, section 8 of the Family Law Reform Act 1969 set a 'medical age of majority' at sixteen enabling such older teenagers to give an effective consent' to treatment. None the less the Court of Appeal held that: 'There can . . . be no doubt that [the court] has power to override the refusal of a minor, whether over the age of sixteen or under that age but *Gillick* competent'. They went on to say that regardless of whether an older child had acquired a right to consent to treatment under sixteen because she was '*Gillick* competent', or at over sixteen because of the operation of the Family Law Reform Act, that child had no right to veto treatment. Parental rights to authorise treatment endured side by side with the child's right until the age of eighteen. If a minor under eighteen refuses treatment, parents can lawfully authorise that treatment if they and the doctors agree that treatment is in the best interests of the minor. Lord Donaldson changed his analogy concerning keyholders (developed in *Re R*) to one relating to flakjackets. He described patient consent as a flakjacket protecting a doctor from being sued for trespass. As long as someone entitled to do so provided the doctor with a flakjacket (consent) he could lawfully go ahead with treatment. Patient autonomy is thus reduced to a mere device for avoiding litigation!

Nurses and older teenagers

A superficial analysis of *Re R* and *Re W* suggests some ludicrous scenarios. A fourteen-year-old who is '*Gillick* competent' can authorise an abortion for herself, yet a seventeen-year-old may be compelled by her parents to terminate a pregnancy? The fifteen-year-old daughter of one of the authors, who could obtain the Pill without her mother's knowledge, can be forced in her own best interests to accept the dreaded fixed brace? The nurse will fear that she will end up 'piggy in the middle' as children, parents and doctors battle over treatment options, but that is unlikely. All the judges in *Re W* stress that while the older teenager has no absolute veto over treatment, objections by such a teenager are to be given great weight. The parental desire for their child to be treated, when the child objects, does not oblige the doctor to treat. The doctor must decide, whether in the light of the child's opposition, treatment will truly benefit. Coercing an unwilling teenager into a forced abortion is likely to do more harm than good. Forcing orthodontic treatment on a resentful fifteen-year-old is likely to be futile.

Re R and *Re W* in effect grant to doctors the right to arbitrate between parents and their older children. The doctor decides whether to accept the child's opposition to treatment or rely on the parents' authorisation of treatment. What is the nurse's role? We would suggest that she should see herself as an advocate for the child-patient and a mediator in the family dispute. The nurse may have a much longer lasting relationship with child and family. She may be better placed to explore the nature of the child's opposition to treatment and to represent the child's objections more coherently both to the parents and professional colleagues.

What about the Children Act?

You may be surprised that so far not much more than passing reference has been made to the Children Act. That Act is crucial when what is at stake is how to protect the welfare of a child at risk of abuse or neglect. Provision is made for social services departments to act swiftly to take a child into care by obtaining an emergency protection order. Where a child's health or injuries provoke doubt about his care, a child assessment order may be sought to compel parents to bring the child for medical examination. Nurses will often be involved in case conferences to decide whether to bring proceedings under the Act. The details of the law protecting children from abuse and neglect would comprise a book of their own.

However, the Children Act is not just about child abuse or the fate of children whose parents separate. It was hailed as representing a new philosophy whereby children's rights and wishes gained new respect. Following the lead of the House of Lords in *Gillick*, parental rights were redefined as parental responsibilities. Children's welfare was expressly stated to take into account children's wishes. Children were given the right to take their own case to court in certain cases. Procedures for resolving disputes were made simpler and more straightforward.

None of the above has in practice much affected the legal principles governing disputes about medical treatment. The following points need to be understood:

1. Either parent, or any other person having parental responsibilities, can authorise treatment of a younger child.
2. Where a court order is sought to require a certain procedure to take place a 'specific issue order' or a 'prohibited steps order' may be applied for under section 8 of the Act, but only if the child is under sixteen.
3. The child could seek leave to obtain a section 8 order for herself or himself.
4. In practice most disputes, whether the child is under or over sixteen, seem to be being dealt with using the 'inherent jurisdiction' of the court.
5. The Act expressly bans any medical examination of a child for the purpose of instituting care proceedings, or seeking an assessment or emergency protection order if a child of 'sufficient understanding' refuses consent.

Yet a judge has held that in exceptional cases the court may bypass the rules and procedures of the Act and order the child to submit where to do so is unequivocally beneficial to him. In *South Glamorgan* v. *X* (1993) Mr Justice Douglas Brown applied the reasoning in *Re R* and *Re W* even to procedures expressly defined by the 1989 Act.

Conclusion

Ethicists and lawyers agree on two issues. Parental rights to determine their children's treatment are not absolute. They are circumscribed by a responsibility to act for the child's benefit and society claims a say in what constitutes such benefit. Autonomy is not acquired overnight but by a gradual process of maturation. Beyond that point ethics and law may to some extent part company. The law denies true autonomy until the age of eighteen. The effect of *Re R* and *Re W* is that in many instances doctors, not parents or children, are left to define the child's best interests. The nurse must struggle to ensure her patient's voice is heard.

10

Caring for vulnerable people

Any person suffering from some form of illness and particularly those removed from their usual environment and admitted to hospital can be considered vulnerable. Even so, there are some groups of individuals who are considered to be especially vulnerable and in some circumstances to require special legal protection. Typically these individuals are those diagnosed as having a mental illness or those with learning difficulties, although children and the elderly are also often vulnerable. In this chapter we address some of the ethical and legal issues that are relevant to the mentally ill, those with learning disabilities and the elderly. The issues relevant to children have been dealt with earlier.

These groups of people will often have diminished autonomy and in addition may be cared for in institutional settings which will further limit their autonomy. Mental illness is often stigmatised in society even though a more liberal approach to caring for such people has been adopted in recent years. The traditional large institutions with extensive grounds typically built on the periphery of towns and cities are no longer considered to be the ideal places to care for mentally ill or those with learning disabilities and many are now cared for in the community with support from community nurses and other services.

Autonomy and the vulnerable patient

The principle of autonomy, that is, the principle that places high value on a person's ability to make their own decisions, is discussed in detail in Chapter Four. We can identify three different groups of vulnerable patients who may have diminished autonomy. Firstly there are those individuals who are unable at present and may never have been able to care for themselves such as those with learning disabilities. Secondly, there are those who become incapable of caring for themselves such as the elderly. These two groups differ from the third group of people, the mentally ill, who may be able to care for themselves in some circumstances, but not in others.

Although these groups of individuals are often recognised as having limited autonomy, it does not follow that they are incapable of making any autonomous decisions at all. People who are not judged competent to consider information given to them with a view to giving informed consent about their treatment or care may be perfectly capable of making some choices. For example, an elderly confused person may have difficulty understanding information given to him about surgery that his doctors advise that he should have, causing him to refuse to give consent. It is quite possible, however, that he will be able to select what clothes he wants to wear and how much sugar he takes in his tea.

There may be other situations when health professionals have to make decisions on behalf of a patient in order to act in the best interests of that patient. Health professionals acting in this way may be behaving in a paternalistic manner, but this may possibly be necessary to protect the patient's best interests. Suppose that a patient with a psychotic mental illness refuses his medication. The nurse knows that the medication is essential to treat the patient's psychosis, but believes that administering it against his will shows a lack of respect for his autonomy. In this situation, the nurse may feel justified in administering the medication, because it is likely that the patient's mental illness is affecting his ability to make rational decisions and give informed consent. Although the nurse is overriding the patient's wishes she is doing so in order to act in his best interests.

Administering essential medication to patients against their wishes appears relatively easy to justify, but what about the patient who refuses to wash or change his clothes; can the nurse justifiably bath him and dress him in clean clothes without his consent? If she does, can the nurse be said to be acting in the patient's best interests? The first thing we need to establish is whose interests are being protected. The nurse may feel that it is better for the patient to be washed and in clean clothes, although for the patient this is of no importance. The nurse cannot be said to be acting in the client's best interests if it is contrary to what he wants and is not likely to cause him any harm. If there is a possibility that the patient may be harmed by being dirty then, as in the previous example, the nurse may be justified in overriding his wishes.

Suppose this patient was admitted to hospital and because of his behaviour was causing distress to other patients and clients on the ward. Clearly the nurse has to consider the interests of all the patients in her care and she would need to balance the wishes of the patient to remain unwashed and dress how he pleases, against the wishes of the other patients on the ward. In this situation, the nurse may feel obliged to bath the patient and change his clothes in order to protect the interests of the other patients and clients in her care.

There is a danger that health professionals caring for vulnerable clients may become so accustomed to making decisions on behalf of their clients that the patients' opinions are never sought even on matters on which they may be able to express a preference. Nurses caring for vulnerable patients will therefore need to be able to assess when clients with diminished autonomy are incapable of making rational choices and recognise other situations when they are competent to decide for themselves. The obvious difficulty lies in how to assess a client's competence.

Informed consent and the vulnerable patient

Vulnerable patients may be judged to be incompetent to give informed consent to a variety of interventions considered necessary and in some cases such a decision will be justified. Under the Mental Health Act 1983, for example, it is not always necessary to obtain informed consent from patients and clients for treatment for their psychiatric disorder. Recent guidelines from the NHS Management Executive indicate that treatment for other illnesses may also be administered to incompetent clients, if such treatment is judged to be in the client's best interests. There are, of course, benefits to this as it allows other forms of treatment and care to be implemented quickly. Suppose someone with schizophrenia is acutely ill with a perforated duodenal ulcer but refuses to give consent to surgery. Unquestionably the patient needs to have the surgery performed, as not doing so would endanger his life. According to the guidelines, the health care professionals would be justified in carrying out the surgery without the consent of the patient if they could show that it was in the client's best interests, which in this case it clearly would be. The alternative would be to say that it was in the patient's best interests to die.

There are, however, more controversial procedures that are more difficult to justify. What about a twenty-year-old woman with learning disabilities who is believed by her family to be sexually active, but who has no understanding of the implications of this? Can she be sterilised if she is judged incompetent to give consent to the surgery? Again, this will depend upon whose interests are being protected, and decisions of this sort rely on others knowing what will be in the best interests of the client, rather than what is in the best interests of the patient's relatives or even the health professionals. The woman may be unable to care for any children she delivered and be dependent upon assistance from her family. It may be argued that it would not be in the woman's best interests to allow her to risk becoming pregnant and that she should be protected from this. Such intervention may be justified if there is no other way of controlling this woman's fertility and it could be shown that by performing the sterilisation her interests would be protected. Later in this chapter we will look again at these issues in a legal context in the case of *F* v. *West Berkshire Health Authority and another*.

The elderly are particularly vulnerable, as they may not be included in decisions regarding their treatment or care, simply because they are elderly, yet they have not been assessed as incompetent to participate. For example, health professionals caring for elderly clients often make decisions about whether the person is to be resuscitated or not should the patient suffer a cardiac arrest. In some instances it is decided that it would not be appropriate to implement the resuscitation procedure and this is recorded in the client's records. A decision of this sort may be made with the best possible motives and it is not considered usual practice to involve the client in the decision-making process, nor inform them of what decision has been made on their behalf.

Clearly there are some patients and clients for whom discussions of this sort would be inappropriate, such as those who are suffering from some form of dementia, but it is unlikely that this will be true for every elderly person. Some patients are well able to make decisions of this sort, and we need to ask why they are not included in the decision-making process. It may be that a patient would be distressed by being asked if they would like to be resuscitated or not and, in effect, asking them may cause them more harm than not doing so. Alternatively, it may be that health professionals are uncomfortable discussing this subject with patients. While this may be understandable, health professionals acting in this way would be protecting their own interests rather than those of the patient. It may be argued that decisions of this sort made on behalf of patients when they could have been consulted is a form of involuntary euthanasia.

Research and the vulnerable patient

As discussed above, there are difficulties in assessing the competence of these patients to make an autonomous decision and give informed consent. As a consequence, if a person is unable to give informed consent, he cannot be considered suitable as a potential research subject. However, it may be argued that there could be exceptions to this. Suppose that someone wants to carry out some research on the effects of art therapy on clients with mental illness. It is impossible to use any research subjects other than those with mental illness, but there are doubts over the clients' ability to give informed consent. It is considered that the results of this research will be of benefit both to those patients participating, and others with similar mental health problems. Can such research be ethical?

One way of answering this is to take a consequentialist view and assess whether the benefits anticipated from the results of this research are greater than the risks of participation. In this example, the physical risks to the client will be minimal, although it may be more difficult to assess the potential emotional or psychological harm. On balance, the risks to the patient appear small in comparison to the anticipated benefits. Of course much would depend on exactly how beneficial the results were considered to be to the participants and others in the future, but if the research is considered to be of value and the risks of participation minimal it may be considered as justified.

There are other situations where it would be more difficult to justify research on vulnerable patients. For example, there is evidence that in the past some vulnerable patients, particularly those in institutions caring for those with learning disabilities, were used as subjects for research that was not only potentially harmful, but with little or no perceived benefits to those involved. Such research cannot be justified and is unethical (for further details see Chapter Eleven).

Advocacy

In its document *Exercising Accountability* the UKCC states its expectation that nurses will accept a role as advocate on behalf of patients and clients. Advocacy in this context means to plead the case of another, or speak out on another person's behalf. This role is arguably of more importance when caring for those groups of patients identified as being particularly vulnerable, as in many instances they will be unable to speak for themselves. The UKCC considers advocacy to be positive and a constructive activity, while acknowledging that there is a potential for conflict. Conflict may arise between professional groups or between the nurse and the patient's relatives over what is to be done in the best interests of the patient when he is unable to voice this himself.

The crucial thing to bear in mind when acting as someone's advocate is that his views are accurately presented, rather than the views of the advocate. Of course, in some circumstances it will not be possible to know exactly what the client would prefer as for example in the recent case of Tony Bland, when a decision was made to stop treating and feeding him because he was in a persistent vegetative state considered to be irreversible. In other circumstances, the advocate may need simply to voice the opinions of clients if they are unable to do so themselves.

Although nurses are in many ways suited to acting as the patient's advocate, the role cannot be claimed exclusively as a nursing one. What would happen for example if someone needed to act as the client's advocate against a decision made by nurses or if other health professionals believe that they are in the best position to act in the client's interests? It may also be unrealistic to assume that a nurse can always act according to the client's preferences, because, as well as having obligations to patients and clients, nurses have obligations to their employers and the professional body, and are bound by legal constraints.

Even amongst groups of patients identified as being especially vulnerable, not all clients will require an advocate, or some may require an advocate in certain situations, but in other circumstances be competent to make their own preferences known. In her assessment of clients, a nurse should be able to identify which clients are likely to need someone to act as their advocate and in what circumstances. The role of advocate, if necessary, can be adopted by the person most appropriate to represent the client according to the circumstances.

Ethically problematic treatment

In some situations nurses may find themselves participating in forms of treatment that they consider to be ethically problematic. One area of controversy for nurses caring for the mentally ill is over the issue of electroconvulsive therapy (ECT). The benefits of ECT have been questioned particularly as it carries with it an element of risk as well as being uncomfortable for the client. In view of this, some nurses have decided to refuse to participate on moral grounds when clients are being given ECT. The limitations on conscientious objection have been discussed in Chapters Three and Eight but in other situations if the nurse considers that the risk to the patient outweighs the benefits then she may be justified in refusing to participate.

Although a nurse may face disciplinary measures from her employing authority for behaving in this way, we may also ask of what benefit this will be to individual patients and clients if they are to receive the treatment anyway. One way of answering this is to say that if enough nurses acted in this way then perhaps the whole question of the benefits of the treatment would be opened up to public debate. In addition, no health professional should be forced to participate in treatment that he or she believes to be detrimental to the well-being of patients and clients, and a nurse could cite clause one of the *Code of Professional Conduct* to support this.

If the patient has given consent to the treatment, then it may be argued that as long as the quality of the information that the patient has been given is sufficient for her to make a truly informed consent then whether she receives the treatment or not is up to her. Difficulties will arise if the nurse considers that the patient has not been given sufficient information or if consent has not been given. Health professionals may find it difficult to accept decisions that a client may make but that is not a sufficient reason to deny her any role in decision-making processes.

The vulnerable patient and the law

Ethical considerations relating to the case of vulnerable patients can be seen to be broadly based. Your obligation as a nurse is to struggle to recognise the autonomy a patient possesses or retains, while at the same time having a proper regard for her welfare. Exploitation of such patients must be guarded against, and on occasion you have to recognise that patients sometimes need to be protected against themselves. The law's focus at present is rather narrower. The Mental Health Act 1983 largely codifies the law governing psychiatric treatment – treatment for mental disorder. The principles defining patients' rights and professional obligations under the Act can be explained relatively simply. But the Act is solely concerned with psychiatric treatment and makes no provision for treatment of physical illness. The legality of routine treatment for everyday ills affecting those with learning difficulties, sterilising women, operating on a hernia suffered by an elderly demented person, all fall to the common law. The law is at present pretty chaotic. It is based roughly on two fairly straightforward questions. Can the patient give a valid consent to authorise treatment? If not, who can act for her, or how else can treatment lawfully be authorised on her behalf?

As we have seen, any physical contact with another is unlawful unless that other has expressly or implicitly authorised the 'touching'. If a patient's mental disability is profound, she may well be unable to give any sort of meaningful consent to treatment. Yet it would be inhumane and ridiculous to say that she could not be treated at all. No one would argue that the elderly patient whose dementia prevents her from consenting to have her ears syringed should simply be left alone for deafness to compound her dementia. In the case of children, the law allows their parents to act on their behalf. If the natural carers, the parents, do not fulfil their responsibilities to the child, the court will intervene. However, once a person is over eighteen no one else can lawfully consent on his behalf. Proxy consent has no legal effect. Next of kin are often asked to sign consent forms on behalf of unconscious or mentally disabled relatives but, in strict law, such forms are meaningless.

The vulnerable patient then, unable to consent for herself, exists in legal limbo. The only statutory provisions relevant to such a case apply in a tiny minority of cases. Section 63 of the Mental Health Act 1983 dispenses with the need to obtain consent for treatment for mental disorder in the case of a patient compulsorily detained under the Act. Very few patients with mental handicap or dementia are so detained. Even if a patient is detained, the Act only allows non-consensual psychiatric treatment. A detained patient may be given antipsychotic drugs against her will, but she cannot be made to have a rotten tooth out. The National Assistance Act 1948 authorises community physicians to remove from home to suitable premises persons suffering from chronic disease or those being aged, infirm or physically incapacitated, who are living in insanitary conditions and are unable to care for themselves. The Act does not authorise actually treating such patients subsequent to their removal from home!

In the vast majority of cases where doubt exists about the autonomy of a vulnerable adult patient, no express authority sanctions treatment. Yet, of course, such patients are treated. Until very recently health professionals and families simply went ahead and did what they believed to be best for the patient. However, as overt paternalism attracted more and more criticism, and as doctors in particular became concerned about litigation, doubt as to the legality and propriety of non-consensual treatment became more widespread. That concern ultimately led to the landmark judgment in the House of Lords in F v. *West Berkshire Health Authority*.

From 1987 onwards a series of cases were referred to the courts, relating to the legality of carrying out abortions and/or sterilisation on women with learning disabilities. In *Re B* (1987) the patient in question was only seventeen. Her case was referred to the Family Division of the High Court. The House of Lords held that parental authority alone was insufficient to authorise such radical, irreversible surgery. But the court could give permission to go ahead with sterilisation where the girl would never acquire the capacity to decide on such matters for herself and sterilisation was in her best interests. In *T* v. *T* a woman of nineteen with profound disabilities, said to have a mental age of two and a half, became pregnant. She was doubly incontinent and had minimal communication skills. Her doctors applied to Mr Justice Wood in the High Court for a declaration that it would be lawful to terminate T's pregnancy and then to sterilise her. The judge found himself in a dilemma. Neither T's mother nor anyone else could consent to the operation on T's behalf. There is no procedure by which guardians able to consent to medical treatment can be appointed by the Court. Any inherent jurisdictional *parens patriae* powers the courts may have had to intervene to protect adults with learning disabilities had lapsed in 1960. All the judge could do was issue a declaration that as T was so mentally impaired as never to be able to consent to treatment, her doctors were justified in 'taking such steps as good medical practice demands'.

A similar set of facts prompted the judgment in the House of Lords in 1989 in *F* v. *West Berkshire HA*. F was thirty-six years old with a mental age of around five to six. She was a voluntary patient in a mental hospital and was believed to have embarked on a sexual relationship with a male patient. The House of Lords granted a declaration stating that F might lawfully be sterilised. Lord Brandon declared: '. . . a doctor can lawfully operate on, or give other treatment to, adult patients who are incapable, for one reason or another, of consenting to his doing so, provided that the operation or other treatment concerned is in the best interests of the patient' (p. 551).

Their lordships made it clear that incompetent adult patients could lawfully receive medical care and treatment. The justification for treatment without consent, according to the House of Lords, rests on the necessity to ensure such patients do receive the treatment their welfare demands.

Health care practitioners therefore have a wide discretion to decide when, and what, treatment is necessary. In such cases the lawfulness of the procedure depends on establishing that what is to be done is in the patient's 'best interests' and is sanctioned by good medical practice.

The law does not formally require that the patient's relatives or carers agree to treatment, or even that they be consulted. Even in the case of radical interventions such as sterilisation it is not mandatory to seek the approval of the court before embarking on surgery. However, the Law Lords strongly advised health professionals, first, that in determining the patient's best interests, all those involved in the care of the patient should be fully consulted, and second, that where irreversible, radical or controversial treatment was proposed the court ought to be approached to give a declaration as to the legality of the procedure. None the less ultimately the judgment about whether and how to proceed rests with the health professionals. It was argued in F that in establishing what constitutes good practice the courts should demand near-unanimity among health professionals as to how best to care for an incompetent patient. That argument was firmly rejected by the House of Lords. The test of good practice is once again the *Bolam* test. The health professional acts lawfully if he or she complies with a practice endorsed by a reasonable body of professional opinion.

Where routine health care is an issue the effect of the judgment in F is this. As long as the professional's purpose is to look after the patient's welfare and she follows an accepted practice she acts lawfully. In effect she acts as the patient's proxy. She decides what to do on behalf of the patient. So if an elderly demented patient needs dental care or cataract surgery, whatever needs to be done can be done. There is unlikely to be any dispute as to what constitutes either the patient's interests or good practice. The problems with F arise where there is genuine disagreement about how best to care for the patient. Should you sterilise women with learning disabilities, or should you protect them from sexual contact? Should you give antibiotics to a patient of eighty-three who has Alzheimer's disease and contracts pneumonia? Those are the sorts of cases where the Law Lords suggest professionals might seek the advice of the court by way of an application for a declaration. But whom do such court proceedings protect? Hopefully it would be the patient, but that may not always be the case. The incentive to persuade health professionals to seek a declaration may well be to protect themselves from any subsequent litigation. Once a court hearing is under way the crucial issues will be whether other professionals (reasonable professional opinion) support what the patient's doctors propose to do, and whether that action can be shown to be in the patient's interests.

Although the series of court cases establishing the legality of non-consensual treatment relates to controversial invasive procedures such as sterilisation, the judgment in F makes it quite clear that the 'best interests' tests apply equally to routine care and all aspects of nursing care. Indeed, they apply to family carers too, ensuring that, as Lord Goff put it, 'the nurse who cares for him, even the relative or friend or neighbour who comes in to look after [the patient], will commit no wrong when he or she touches his body' (p. 564).

As we suggested earlier when routine treatment is clearly aimed at relieving suffering or preventing deterioration in health, no problem arises in determining the patient's interests. Lord Bridge declared that it was: 'axiomatic that treatment which is necessary to preserve the life, health or well-being of the patient may lawfully be given' (p. 548). Alas, that treatment is necessary for these purposes may sometimes be less than clear. Consider this example. An elderly patient in a elderly care unit refuses to co-operate in being washed or changing his underpants, or taking medication to help him sleep. He stinks and wanders the ward at night. Washing and changing him, and ensuring a good night's sleep are all desirable, but are they necessary? The interests of everybody else in the ward are served by improving his hygiene and sleep pattern, but strictly speaking the law requires you to consider only that patient's individual interests. Another difficult issue arises where patients tend to wander. Can you justify locking the doors of an elderly care unit because a patient might wander out of the grounds of the hospital on to a main road? Can you prevent young women with learning disabilities from coming into contact with men who may exploit them? Even if the women have been sterilised, they are still at risk of disease or exploitation. You have to ask whether restraint is truly necessary in their interest? Or is the answer that restraint is in your interests, to make your job as a carer easier and protect yourself if the patient comes to harm?

The formulation used to justify non-consensual treatment in *F* raises grave doubts about the legality of clinical research involving incompetent patients. Therapeutic research may be lawful if you can establish that the chance of benefit to the patient is sufficient to render his participation in research in his 'best interests'. Non-therapeutic research where no conceivable benefit will accrue to the patient cannot be classified as treatment in the subject's best interests. Wherever researchers seek to carry out research on an incompetent patient posing a risk of harm, discomfort or distress to the patient, the legality of such research must be considered extremely dubious to say the least.

But who is competent?

In the series of cases which have gone to the English courts to establish the legality of treatment of incompetent patients, the inability of the patient to consent for herself (her incompetence) has been taken for granted. Criteria defining the degree of intelligence and understanding needed to be competent have not been clearly declared. One matter, though, is clear. In England capacity to consent, i.e. competence, relates very specifically to the procedure or transaction in question. People are not placed in rigid categories, competent to consent to every procedure or incompetent in every aspect of life. In law there are no fixed criteria by which to assess competence. The question asked is whether a person possesses the required degree of understanding to proceed with the particular enterprise or transaction. So, for example, requisite degree of understanding may vary according to whether the person is entering into a contract, getting married or making a will. The case of *In the Estate of Park* (1954) illustrates the elusive nature of the concept of competence in English law. Mr Park was an elderly man who, after suffering a severe stroke, married his second wife one morning and that afternoon executed a new will. He died shortly afterwards. His family challenged the validity of the marriage and his widow challenged the will. The court found him to have been mentally competent to marry, but to lack sufficient mental capacity to make a will. A much lower level of understanding was required to consent to marriage!

So, how will the courts regard consent to medical treatment? From *Chatterton* v. *Gerson* you will know that for a patient's consent to be valid, the patient need only be informed in broad terms about the nature and purpose of the treatment intended. Logically it would appear that is all he need understand. Therefore the level of understanding at which a patient is legally competent to give his own consent to treatment is fairly low. Without doubt many patients with some degree of mental illness or learning disability possess the requisite minimal level of competence to authorise their own treatment. A psychiatric illness or condition is not on its own sufficient grounds to justify compulsory treatment. But what if, although understanding enough to authorise the treatment, the patient refuses to give consent? For example, an elderly confused patient refuses dental treatment because he fears the pain: the short-term preference for avoiding pain outweighing the long-term advantages of treatment.

Assuming I am fully competent, if I am diagnosed tomorrow as suffering from a physical illness which will be terminal unless treated, no one can force me to undergo that treatment. Whatever the nature of my illness, I may decline to agree to treatment and I am not obliged to justify my decision. Thousands of people motivated by irrational fear avoid the dentist. No one has as yet proposed compulsory dental care for adults. Yet the current relatively low threshold for competence prompts concern that vulnerable patients will decline, and thus not receive the treatment, they need. But who is to define need? In the case of *Re C* (1994), a patient with chronic schizophrenia also suffered from diabetes. As is so often the case with diabetics he began to suffer problems with his foot and there was a fear that gangrene would develop. His doctors wanted to amputate his lower leg. C applied to the court for an order that neither now nor in the future should doctors operate to amputate his limb without his express consent. The judge found that despite his mental disorder, C understood the nature and consequences of the proposed surgery. He could no more be forced to comply than you could. English law adopts a functional test of competence. Do you comprehend what you are being asked or agree to? That the outcome may be one doctors, nurses, and relatives disagree with should not be relevant.

Unfortunately outcomes are not the only difficulties if you adopt a low threshold of competence. In practice, few vulnerable patients will disagree with the health professionals caring for them. Most will simply acquiesce. The nurse has a special responsibility to try and ensure that, as far as humanly possible, the vulnerable patient has a real opportunity to make his own decision. Simple straightforward language should be used and time should be taken for the information to sink in. Relatives and friends can be called in to help the patient decide. Vulnerable patients should never be steam-rollered into signing a consent form.

Proposals for reform

The Law Commission has undertaken an extensive review of the law relating to mentally incapacitated patients. Their concern has been much wider than the particular issue of consent to health care treatment. The law relating to management of an incompetent patient's property and money, and who is responsible for his general welfare is just as crucial to the individual. In relation to health care the reforms so far proposed centre on these areas.

1. A new jurisdiction should be granted to the courts akin to the inherent jurisdiction in relation to children. The courts would become the final arbiter in disputes concerning the care of vulnerable patients.
2. Resort to the courts in cases of especial difficulty or controversy would be mandatory, not a procedure that health professionals could choose to invoke if they thought it necessary.
3. Statutory provision would be made to authorise routine treatment and protection granted to professionals who act in good faith.
4. In certain circumstances the law would change to allow a carer or relative to act as the patient's proxy, as his guardian, so to speak. This could happen in two ways. The proxy could be chosen by the court. Or where a patient has in his lifetime been competent, he could, in advance of incompetence resulting from age or disease, nominate his own proxy by way of a durable power of attorney for health care.

The Law Commission also addressed itself to the definition of competence and recommended broadly that we retain the current functional test of competence, but with two important qualifications. First, if a patient is unable to communicate, and all reasonable efforts to establish communication with the patient have failed, he should be treated as incompetent. Second, even where a patient has the necessary understanding and intelligence to comprehend what is proposed to him, he should be deemed incompetent if he lacks the capacity to make a 'true choice'.

At the time of writing, the Law Commission's own final proposals have not yet emerged. Whether those proposals will be accepted and acted on by the Government is uncertain. You should give particular thought to the following questions. The Law Commission rejected any automatic right for family members to act as proxy for adult patients. By inserting into the definition of competence the notion of 'true choice', it becomes possible to override refusal of treatment by patients who fully understand the nature of treatment. The elderly lady whose fear of the dentist is such that she refuses to have her abscessed tooth removed may be compelled to do so. The anorexic girl whose disease has deprived her of the ability to see her body as it is rather than as she perceives it will be able to be treated lawfully regardless of whether she is sixteen or nineteen. Tragic outcomes will be avoided, but at what cost to autonomy?

Treatment for mental disorder

The law becomes rather more straightforward if the question of issue concerns psychiatric treatment. The Mental Health Act 1983 regulates the in-patient treatment of both voluntary (informal) and involuntary (detained or formal) patients. The Act created the Mental Health Commission which was designed to provide an additional level of protection for psychiatric patients. The Commission has extensive powers to inspect and supervise care in mental hospitals. The policy on which the Act rests is a balancing operation designed to protect the welfare and rights of patients while at the same time minimising the risk patients pose either to others or themselves. You must also bear in mind that only the very minimum number of patients are, and should be, detained in hospital, and deprived of their liberty altogether. And, of course, current Government policy seeks to limit the number of in-patients in hospital overall preferring to promote care in the community.

Informal (voluntary) treatment is regulated by section 131 of the Act which provides that patients may be admitted to hospital for psychiatric treatment without any order being made and remain free to leave whenever they choose. Informal patients retain the right to refuse treatment. They have the same access to the courts as any other person. The legal status of a voluntary mentally ill patient is therefore very similar to that of a patient in any other hospital in terms of perceived rights and duties owed. This does not necessarily mean that they are actually treated in the same way. Such patients' consent may not always be sought in practice before minor or routine procedures. They may often not be in a position to understand the information provided in order to give effective consent. They may well be prepared simply to acquiesce in whatever their doctors propose.

The most important difference between informal patients in mental hospitals and others receiving 'ordinary care' is that an informal patient's status in a psychiatric hospital may be changed to that of compulsory detention (s.5(1)). The 'doctor in charge' of the patient may effect that change of status if she thinks that 'an application ought to be made' for compulsory admission (s.5(2)), but the patient may only be detained in this manner for seventy-two hours. A nurse may also prevent a patient leaving hospital if he believes it is immediately necessary and if it is not immediately practicable to secure the attendance of the doctor in charge or her delegate (s.5(4)). In this case the patient may only be detained for six hours or until a doctor is able to attend. This can mean that if an informal patient is not submissive the 'threat' of detention can be invoked to secure compliance with the professional's wishes.

Part II of the Act provides for the compulsory detention in hospital of certain mentally disordered patients – what is colloquially referred to as 'sectioning a patient'. Compulsory admission may be enforced on a person in three ways: admission for assessment under section 2; emergency admission under section 4; admission for treatment under section 3.

In the case of admission for assessment under section 2, the patient's nearest relative or an approved social worker may make an application for such admission. The applicant must have seen the patient within the last fourteen days and the application must be endorsed by two registered medical practitioners (one of whom must be qualified in psychiatry). The applicant is responsible for getting the patient to hospital and reasonable use of force is permissible. The grounds for admission under section 2 are that the patient firstly is suffering from mental disorder of a nature warranting his detention in hospital, at least for a limited period, and, secondly, ought to be so detained in the interests of his own health or safety, or to protect others. Admission for the assessment authorises the patient's detention for twenty-eight days. For further detention an application for admission for treatment must be made.

Emergency admissions are regulated by section 4. A single doctor may recommend such an admission which is valid for seventy-two hours. The doctor does not have to be a specialist in mental illness, but if possible she must have known the patient beforehand and must have seen the patient within the previous twenty-four hours. Emergency admission may be converted to admission for assessment (twenty-eight days) by obtaining an additional opinion from a mental illness specialist.

Admission for treatment under section 3 allows for longer-term compulsory detention. The application procedures are similar to those for assessment but in this case the nearest relative must be consulted when admission is being sought by a social worker. If the relative objects, court authority will be needed. If the application is successful, admission for treatment authorises detention for an initial period of six months. Section 3 provides that the application must be based on the grounds that the patient:

(a) is suffering from mental illness, severe mental impairment, psychopathic disorder or mental impairment and his mental disorder is of a nature or degree which makes it appropriate for him to receive treatment in a mental hospital; and

(b) in the case of psychopathic disorder or mental impairment, such treatment is likely to alleviate or prevent a deterioration in his conditions; and

(c) it is necessary for the health and safety of the patient or for the protection of other persons that he should receive such treatment and it cannot be provided unless he is detained under this section.

Because the six-month period is renewable, detention under section 3 may last indefinitely. In the event of aggrieved patients bringing proceedings against those responsible for their detention, section 139 states: 'No person shall be liable ... to any civil or criminal proceedings ... in respect of any act purporting to be done in pursuance of this Act ... unless the act was done in bad faith or without reasonable care.' Furthermore, in order to bring proceedings alleging bad faith or negligence, permission has to be obtained from the High Court.

The powers granted under the Act can thus be seen to be pretty draconian, so what are the conditions that may result in compulsory detention? Strangely enough, 'mental illness' is nowhere defined in the Act. Definition and diagnosis of such illness are entrusted to the psychiatrists. 'Severe mental impairment' is defined as 'a state of arrested or incomplete development of mind which includes severe impairment of intelligence and social functioning'. Psychopathic disorder is self-defining. 'Mental impairment' is defined in terms similar to severe mental impairment save that the relative impairment of intelligence and social functioning need not be severe, only significant. A diagnosis of mental illness is sufficient on its own to warrant detention under the Act. In other cases of severe mental impairment, mental impairment or psychopathic disorder, evidence of 'abnormally aggressive or seriously irresponsible behaviour' must be present. If a patient suffers from simple mental impairment or psychopathic disorder, compulsory detention must be shown to be likely to result in treatment that will alleviate, or at least prevent deterioration in, the patient's condition. Finally, in every instance it must be demonstrated that treatment cannot be provided except by means of compulsory detention. Mentally ill patients or those with learning disabilities cannot simply be shut away out of sight.

The stringent safeguards laid down before a patient can be compulsorily detained mean that in reality very few patients, other than those who are actively mentally ill, are formally detained in hospital. That large group of especially vulnerable patients who suffer from varying degrees of mental disability are unlikely to be candidates for formal admission to hospital. First, few such patients do demonstrate abnormally aggressive or seriously irresponsible behaviour. Second, their condition is unlikely to be treatable and whatever care they need can be provided outside the boundaries of a secure mental hospital. And finally, of course, current policy dictates that wherever possible patients should be cared for in the community and not in hospital regardless of whether the patient is in hospital as an informal or detained patient.

Where patients are treated in hospital, however, you should note that for once the role of the nurse as a key professional in the overall care and management of patients is expressly recognised. 'Medical treatment' is defined to include nursing care, habilitation and rehabilitation under medical supervision. Nurses as we saw are empowered by section 5 of the Act to detain informal patients for up to six hours where it is necessary to do so to protect the patient or others and prevent him leaving the hospital, and where it is not practicable for a doctor to attend the patient immediately to assess his condition. Where the powers granted under Part IV of the Act in relation to compulsory and/or radical treatment come into play, the patient's nurse must be consulted before ECT is given or psychosurgery administered. Such powers granted to the nurse enhance her professional status in the health care team. They also bring additional responsibilities and because of their coercive nature can trigger conflict between the nurse's role as advocate and the managerial role the Mental Health Act assigns to her. Most psychiatric hospitals have drawn up further guidance to assist nursing staff in the exercise of their duties. Further advice can be found in the Royal College of Nursing document *Seclusion and Restraint in Hospitals and Units for the Mentally Disordered.*

Compulsory treatment under the Mental Health Act

Where patients are formally detained in hospital, Part IV of the Mental Health Act 1983 allows for compulsory treatment of such patients. Section 63 provides the following: 'The consent of a patient shall not be required for any medical treatment given to him of the mental disorder from which he is suffering, not being treatment given within section 57 or 58 [of the Act].' Never forget that section 63 only applies to detained patients. It cannot be used on voluntary patients, or on an out-patient basis. Nor can a patient be brought into hospital, detained and immediately released on licence once he has been given his medication. If he does not need to be detained in hospital, detention cannot be used as a pretext for compulsory treatment in the community. Moreover, section 63 only authorises routine psychiatric treatment and sections 57 and 58 provide safeguards for patients against more draconian therapies.

Section 57 applies to all patients and not just detained patients. Any form of psychosurgery, for example, lobotomy, and any surgical implantation of hormones to reduce male sexual drive is unlawful unless first, the patient consents and secondly, an independent doctor (appointed by the Mental Health Commission) certifies that (a) the patient is capable of understanding the nature and purpose of the treatment proposed and its likely effects; and (b) the treatment is likely to benefit the patient. The Commission acts as a watchdog for patients' interests.

Section 58 applies to detained patients only. Electroconvulsive therapy and any long-term medication (administered for longer than three months) are authorised only if either (a) the patient consents and a doctor certifies that he is competent to do so or (b) an independent medical practitioner certifies that the patient is not competent or has refused to consent, but that none the less 'having regard to the likelihood of [the treatment] alleviating or preventing a deterioration of his condition the treatment should be given'.

The formula for non-consensual treatment proffered by the Mental Health Act is quite simple. Decisions as to routine treatment are made by health care workers. The more serious the proposed treatment, the greater are the safeguards provided for the patient by way of independent review of the initial professional's judgment. But the powers under the Act are only available once a patient has been 'sectioned'. In effect, he has to be 'locked up' before he can be treated.

The Department of Health is currently reviewing the question of whether patients can be forced to accept treatment outside hospital. The impetus for the review was accelerated by the Ben Silcock affair and concern about the number of mentally ill people and those with learning disabilities who are now expected to live in the community. One proposal is based on the idea of supervision orders which would require patients to report to their doctor or community psychiatric nurse. These practitioners would have the power to readmit the patient if he or she failed to report or where there was concern that a discharged patient might suffer a relapse. The problem with such orders is, of course, the fact that they will rely heavily on professional opinion and unless clear guidelines are given as to how the power should be used, patients may be no better off.

Ill, old and alone?

The law at the moment, because it focuses almost exclusively on the narrow question of consent to treatment, makes little or no distinction between the various categories of vulnerable patients. It does not matter whether the person in question cannot authorise treatment for himself because he was afflicted from birth by mental disability, or has suffered devastating brain injuries in an accident, or once having been entirely competent, is now suffering from senile dementia. As long as the key legal question is consent to treatment, the law only has a role to play when the attention of a health professional has been drawn to a patient's need and a specific decision must be made as to how to proceed. As the twentieth century comes to an end increased life expectancy creates an ever-growing population of very elderly people, a proportion of whom succumb to some form of senile dementia and all of whom will be to a greater or lesser extent vulnerable as age limits their physical, if not mental, capabilities. The media carry regular reports of sick elderly people found alone at home in miserable conditions. Disturbing reports of elderly abuse by families and carers of elderly people who do not live alone are becoming more common. The law today is reactive. Should it become more proactive? Nurses working in the community will often be the professionals who first discover the plight of a neglected elderly person, or indeed any other category of vulnerable patient. What action can they take?

The National Health Service and Community Care Act 1990 gives local authorities primary responsibility for co-ordinating community care needs and services. The nurse can now contact the appropriate authorities and start a process which should lead to an investigation of the patient's circumstances and an offer of appropriate care at home or in residential accommodation. However, any positive action requires firstly, the willingness of the local authority to provide adequate resources to fund the care required and secondly, the co-operation of the patient and his family. If a patient refuses help or a family rejects 'interference' there is little that the nurse or anyone else can do at present. Should professionals be given coercive powers to protect elderly patients in the community for 'their own good'?

One such coercive power already exists. Elderly, infirm or incapacitated patients can be removed from their homes under section 47 of the National Assistance Act 1948 (as amended by the National Assistance (Amendment) Act of 1951). An application can be made by a community physician to a magistrate for the person's removal to suitable premises. Few community physicians today are ready to invoke these provisions. The Law Commission in their proposals for law reform have suggested that new legislative powers should become available to protect vulnerable adults. Local social service authorities would be empowered to investigate any report that 'a person is incapacitated, mentally disordered or vulnerable and is suffering or is likely to suffer serious harm [or serious exploitation]'. Consequential powers would enforce access to the person and allow the authority to apply for an emergency protection order to remove that person from home.

None of these powers could be used save when the individual in question suffered from mental disorder (as defined by the Mental Health Act 1983) and lacked capacity to act for himself (i.e. was not competent).

Were these proposals to be acted on they would have the following effect. When a nurse came upon a patient alone and incapable of making any sort of decision for himself, local social services authorities would have formal powers to intervene. Where a patient was not feeding himself, not washing, and no longer able to see why he should do these things, steps could be taken to protect him from himself. If a nurse suspected an elderly patient's bruises were inflicted by an over-burdened son who lost his temper while toileting his mother, or a daughter who was just plain bad, the circumstances could be investigated and this patient removed into adequate care. However, a more likely scenario perhaps is this. A cantankerous patient lives alone in a filthy house with several cats. She will not take the medication which has been prescribed. Sometimes she opens the door to meals on wheels. Sometimes she lets you dress her leg ulcer. Sometimes she simply refuses to answer the door. She knows perfectly well what she is doing. She prefers to live her own life, thank you. Nothing in the Law Commissions's proposals for reform will authorise forcing such a patient to accept help 'for her own good'.

Conclusion

The vulnerable patient poses a difficult challenge to nurses. Reconciling an obligation to protect whatever degree of autonomy the patient enjoys with a responsibility to promote the patient's welfare will never be easy. The law now empowers health professionals to act to protect seriously disturbed and dangerous patients from harming themselves or others. It prescribes, in relation to that tiny minority of formally detained patients, conditions under which autonomy may be overridden. The law authorises the nurse to do what is required to promote the welfare of the patient whose illness or condition deprives him of all ability to act for himself. The Law Commission's proposals will clarify and strengthen the position of the professional in such circumstances. The law offers no help in dealing with the patient who can, but who will not, help himself. The likelihood is that it will not and should not. It is all too easy to say that the very elderly or mentally disabled patient is incompetent and needs 'looking after'. You must be careful not automatically to equate age or mental disability with incompetence. Neither condition necessarily robs a person of all autonomy. Respect for that person requires that you persist in negotiation with him so that together you can reach decisions which best maximise his welfare in every sense. A clean room in a residential home and three meals a day are not necessarily better for him than a crumbling flat filled with his own possessions and the company of an equally elderly, even dirty, dog. Ultimately, on occasion you have to accept that you are unable to help others to help themselves.

11

Nurses and clinical research

Clinical research is an integral part of modern health care. Improvements in treatment require that new techniques and new medicine be tested and evaluated. Without research many of the advances in medicine which have resulted in, amongst other things, greatly increased success rates in the treatment of childhood cancers, safer surgery and better means for wound healing would never have happened. Doing research has always been a major part of a doctor's career. Now research can be equally important for the nurse. She needs to be seen to be developing her discipline and nursing research helps validate her professional status. However, health professionals, unlike some other groups, can often only pursue valuable research by using as their 'research tool' other people, both patients and altruistic volunteers. And the use of fellow humans in research poses an immediate ethical dilemma. The interests of medical science, and of the health professional carrying out research, may conflict with the welfare interests of the research subjects. The fundamental question for ethicists and lawyers posed by clinical research is how to reconcile the scientific imperative to acquire new knowledge for the benefit of the profession and the wider community with the subject's right to autonomy and his general well-being. The atrocities committed in the name of medicine by Japanese and Nazi doctors in the Second World War graphically highlight the horrors that unrestricted and unethical research can lead to.

As a nurse you may find yourself involved in research in a number of ways. You may undertake a research project of your own. Examples of nursing research include investigation into which method of treatment has greatest success for children with minor scalds, research into the after-care of elderly patients and examinations of methods of reducing incontinence in the very elderly confused patient. You may be asked to participate in research either by answering questionnaires and suchlike or 'volunteering' to be a guinea pig for a new drug. Or you may be involved in nursing and caring for patients and subjects enrolled in trials being undertaken by medical staff. The ethical imperative is to ensure that any research involving human beings is properly monitored to protect the rights of the subjects and prevent unjustifiable physical, psychological or emotional harm to them. Many of the problems research may pose are dealt with earlier. Did the subject give an adequate consent to participate in the research? If you believe a research trial is unethical, can you – should you – blow the whistle on the researchers? In this chapter we look at what additional safeguards are needed in the context of clinical research.

Clinical research is often divided into two categories, therapeutic and non-therapeutic research. In therapeutic research, while one of the aims of the research is to acquire new knowledge, the researcher also has reason to hope that the novel therapy under trial will benefit the patient. Suppose a new anti-hypertensive drug is developed and animal trials suggest that it is more effective than existing medication. If Dr X asks patient Y to enrol in the trial of the new drug he intends to gain valuable information to attain the research goals of the trial but he also hopes that the trial will have therapeutic benefit for patient Y. In non-therapeutic research acquisition of knowledge is the only aim of the trial. The subject is asked to undergo certain procedures to benefit the development of medicine but can hope to gain no personal benefit to his own health. Non-therapeutic research can involve fairly minor procedures such as providing blood samples for analysis, or it can have major implications for subjects. A company may want to test a new drug for its effect on liver function, or estimate the safety and efficiency of a new anaesthetic. Students are often asked to volunteer for non-therapeutic trials, and they may be offered money for their pains.

Another way of dividing clinical research into categories is to distinguish between invasive and non-invasive research. Invasive research involves some actual physical contact with the patient or subject, for example, taking blood or injecting a drug intravenously. Non-invasive research avoids such contact. It may involve questionnaires or psychological investigation. The distinction between invasive and non-invasive research is crucial in a legal context. Ethically, remember that non-invasive research can be as distressing and invasive of privacy as any other research project. Imagine that you want to evaluate the link between cervical cancer and sexual practices. The questions you may want to ask subjects and the fears you may provoke could do a lot more harm than a simple venepuncture.

Ethical consideration and research

At the heart of many of the ethical considerations prompted by clinical research lies a simple question. Is the risk to the research subject justified by the potential benefit likely to derive from the research? In every proposal to carry out research a risk/benefit analysis must be attempted. Benefit may take diverse forms. The legitimate aim of research is to add to the body of knowledge in order to improve health care for all of us, but researchers may have motives for carrying out research which fall short of this ideal. Perhaps the question that should really be addressed is, for what purpose is the research being undertaken? Undertaking research is now an important part of the career structure of doctors and nurses. Nurses are often required to undertake a piece of research as part of a course and the publication of research is seen to be prestigious. Research can bring fame and financial reward to the researcher, so in assessing whether research is ethical or not the risks and benefits to both the participant and the researcher need to be considered.

As a general rule, research should only be carried out if the likely benefits to the individual taking part in the research and/or to society as a whole far outweigh the risks of participation. Suppose a nurse forms a hypothesis relating to the definitive cause of pressure sores but in order to prove that hypothesis, she needs to undertake a piece of research. She is aware that research findings will be advantageous to her career and this is her true motivation for wanting to carry out the research. Her chosen method, however, will not involve any physical, psychological or emotional harm to the participants. She merely observes and records patients' histories and conditions. That the researcher is carrying out the research mainly because of self-interest does not necessarily make it ethically problematic. The participants will not be harmed in any way, and they and many others will benefit as a result of this research despite the fact that this is not the researcher's exclusive aim.

Change the example just a little. Suppose that instead of the above harmless research method, to find the definitive cause of pressure sores, participants have to be given electric shocks which are both painful and potentially dangerous. In this situation the risk to the participants is substantial and the researcher would need to assess whether the degree of risk and discomfort was outweighed by the benefits of the results of the research. The researcher acting in self-interest may feel that the benefits are significant both to herself and to society as a whole but the individual participants subjected to a painful and dangerous procedure would probably not agree!

Assessing physical harm in many circumstances is not difficult. The same cannot be said for assessing psychological or emotional harm. This is of particular relevance in nursing research because the diverse nature of the discipline of nursing requires a variety of research methodologies. Just being observed or questioned may make a participant anxious and so be detrimental to his well-being. Because of the difficulties of assessing risk benefit analysis, many professional and regulatory institutions have published ethical codes and guidelines in an attempt to exercise some form of control over research.

Ethical codes and guidelines

The first modern attempt to devise a code of ethics to regulate medical research was provoked by the atrocities committed by Nazi doctors who were later condemned as war criminals. Research carried out by doctors for the benefit of the German armed forces included freezing and high altitude experiments, deliberate infection with malaria, tetanus and gas gangrene, testing the effectiveness of sulphonamides, and investigating the effects of various poisons. These experiments were designed to improve the fighting techniques of the German armed forces as well as improving treatments for diseases commonly contracted as a result of warfare. The experiments were carried out on prisoners. These so-called prisoners were not fairly tried and convicted criminals but people whose only 'crimes' were to be members of social and ethnic groups considered undesirable by the Third Reich. Because of their status, it was not considered necessary to obtain their consent to participate in experiments which often resulted in the death of the participant.

After the war, in 1949, such research methods were condemned and ten principles were identified as essential for the regulation of research. These ten principles became known as the Nuremberg Code. In 1964 the Nuremberg Code was supplemented and expanded by the Declaration of Helsinki promulgated by the World Health Organisation, which was subsequently amended in 1964 and 1983. The first guidelines for nursing research were published by the American Nurses Association in 1968 and since then other guidelines have been published in Canada, New Zealand and by the Royal College of Nursing in this country. These guidelines are similar in substance and address the following issues.

1. The research must make a substantial contribution to the body of nursing knowledge.
2. Emphasis must be placed on the quality of information given to a potential participant to enable them to give their informed consent.
3. The risks of participation must be outweighed by the benefits to the individual and preferably to society as a whole.
4. Consideration must be given to the participants' well-being and the avoidance of physical, psychological or emotional harm.
5. Confidentiality must be respected.
6. The research should only be carried out by those qualified to do so.
7. Participants must be free to withdraw from the research at any time should they request to do so.
8. Potential participants should not be subjected to any form of coercion to consent.
9. Research should only be carried out on vulnerable people such as pregnant women, children or the mentally ill when there are no other alternatives.

As far as research by doctors is concerned, the Royal Colleges of Medicine publish guidance on research and the guidelines devised by the Royal College of Physicians constitute the medical 'gold standard'. Government direction on clinical research is found in the 1991 guidelines published by the Department of Health. Ethical codes and guidelines serve two purposes, firstly, to protect the rights of participants and secondly, to outline the obligations of the researcher, but in practice there are certain limitations to their usefulness.

Limitations of ethical codes and guidelines

The main limitation of any ethical codes or guidelines is that they are exactly as their name suggests, guidelines, and are not directly enforceable by law, so a high level of personal integrity is required of the researcher. Also, as previously discussed, there are difficulties in assessing exactly what constitutes physical, psychological and emotional harm.

Individuals must not be coerced into agreeing to participate in research and should be free to withdraw at any time they wish to do so. In practice, this may be difficult to achieve. A patient or client may feel that if he does not agree to participate in research it may affect the care he is given and that he may as a result receive some inferior treatment. Patients and clients may not want to be viewed as being unhelpful and non-compliant. This is of particular relevance if the researchers are involved in their treatment and care in some other way.

It may seem trite to say that the researcher should possess the necessary skills and qualifications to undertake the research, but this is not always the case. Some courses undertaken by nurses require them to carry out research, but their research skills and the time available are usually limited. As a result, the research is not being carried out by someone qualified to do so nor is it likely to make a significant contribution to the body of nursing knowledge. This is not to say that such research is of no value, but if the aim is to enable the student to acquire fundamental research skills, then other educational activities may provide these without actually undertaking research on patients.

Ethical codes and guidelines are also limited in the guidance they provide for funding research. Research is an expensive activity and the funding of research can raise ethical questions, particularly if funds are obtained from manufacturers to carry out research on their products. Suppose that funding is obtained from manufacturer A for research on the efficacy of their wound care product against the dressing produced by manufacturer B. A may not agree to the publication of the research findings if their product is shown to be less effective. It is not ethically problematic to receive funding from companies and manufacturers to undertake research, but the researchers must not be influenced by the source of the funding in any way, and must ensure that they are free to publish their findings irrespective of the results. Many of the ethical problems encountered in research relate to the issue of informed consent. Consent to treatment has been discussed in Chapter Four, but the subject is of particular relevance for participants in randomised controlled trials.

Randomised controlled trials

A great deal of controversy about informed consent revolves around the issue of randomised clinical trials. Obviously, before any patient is enrolled in any clinical trial, he should be given a full explanation of what will be done to him, what risks to his health are foreseen and what the research seeks to achieve. But in randomised trials it may be impossible to give the patient that full explanation because of the very nature of these sorts of trials. The researcher will not know exactly what risks confront any individual patient. Randomised trials involve allocating patients to groups on a random basis in order to compare treatments. The randomisation will often be 'blind' in the sense that the researcher is unaware which patient is in which group so that her judgment on the efficacy of a particular treatment is not distorted by preconceptions about the efficacy of the trial drug. As the researcher will not know that, say, X is receiving the new drug she cannot fully explain the implications of the trial to X. And consent is not the only difficulty with randomised trials.

Suppose that you want to test the effectiveness of a new antibiotic. You decide that the patients will be divided into three groups, one of which will get the new antibiotic, one of which will receive Ampicillin, which is a known effective antibiotic, and the third group will get a placebo. You inform all patients of the type of research that you are engaged in and explain that they will be allocated one of the three 'treatments', but neither they nor you will know which one it is. If an adequate explanation is given to the patients about this trial, is it likely that many would consent to entering it, as one group is to be denied effective treatment for their illness? If all the patients you speak to do consent to enter the trial, then perhaps others may be justified in doubting that you have been truthful in your explanation.

A further ethical difficulty arises in this sort of trial when some of the participants are denied what is considered to be effective treatment for their illness. Arguably, then, trials can only be justified if doubt exists as to which of two or more treatments is the most effective or to test the efficacy of a new treatment. So you could justify carrying out the clinical trial on the new antibiotic as long as you split the patients into only two groups, one of which would receive the new drug and one Ampicillin. By not using a placebo you are not withholding a recognised form of treatment from any patients.

Open neural tube defects and the use of vitamins

Problems arise in randomised control trials if you are perceived to be withholding an effective treatment. A controversial example of such an ethical dilemma is illustrated by the following case. In 1976 R. W. Smithells, Professor of Paediatrics at Leeds University, published a paper suggesting that blood levels of certain vitamins were lower on average amongst women who later gave birth to babies with neural tube defects such as anencephaly and spina bifida. The obvious conclusion drawn from Professor Smithells' paper was that women who had previously given birth to a child with a neural tube defect should be given vitamin supplements.

Over the next six years, several trials were conducted by Professor Smithells and others and speculation arose as to whether the use of preconceptual vitamin supplementation was effective or not in minimising the incident of such birth defects. Criticism of these trials included the contention that the women participating were not selected at random, a bias in the results was shown and that the numbers were too low to be statistically significant.

The Medical Research Council decided to conduct a multicentre randomised controlled trial to attempt to discover how effective this treatment was, but a storm of protest erupted. Groups of objectors stated that although there might not be complete proof of the efficacy of the vitamins, there was strong evidence to suggest that treatment was effective. As a consequence they argued that it would be unethical to conduct a randomised trial as some women who had previously given birth to a baby with a neural tube defect would be denied the vitamin supplements.

This was an interesting case as the central issue was highly emotive. Everyone would agree that to give birth to a baby with a neural tube defect should be prevented if at all possible, and to deny a possible preventative measure to women at risk seems unnecessarily cruel. The vitamin supplements used were unlikely to have adverse effects on the women who took them even if they in fact did little good. None the less the vitamin 'affair' illustrates the argument that can be used to justify a trial that does of necessity deny treatment to some participants. It goes like this. It is unethical to employ a treatment not proved to be effective. The only means of proving effect is to test the treatment against a placebo. Only if the treatment group shows better results than the placebo group can you know that the treatment, rather than other unrelated factors, is producing the effect you desire. Thus some women should be left at risk in the vitamin trial so all women at a later stage could enjoy a proven benefit.

Research ethics committees

Codes of practice and informed debate on the ethics of clinical trials are all very well, but how can you ensure compliance with ethical principles?

In 1967 M. H. Pappworth published an influential book entitled *Human Guinea Pigs*. In this book Pappworth gave details of hundreds of experiments which he considered to be unethical, most of which had been carried out in the United States and the United Kingdom. Despite the existence of the Declaration of Helsinki, Pappworth argued for research to be more strictly controlled and suggested that ethics committees with at least one lay member should be set up to review research proposals and be legally accountable to the General Medical Council. In the same year, the Royal College of Physicians also published a report on this subject echoing Pappworth's recommendations for reviewing research proposals. As a consequence, many hospitals did set up research ethics committees and in 1973 the Royal College of Physicians at the request of the DHSS made similar recommendations about the regulation of research. In 1975 the DHSS published a circular confirming the RCP recommendations. However, the proposals still had no statutory force. Consequently, although it was recommended that hospitals set up ethics committees with at least one lay member to review research proposals, they were under no legal obligation to do so.

In 1991, after much criticism of the actual working practices of ethics committees, the Department of Health published new guidelines on Local Research Ethics Committees (LREC) which came into effect in February 1992. The Department of Health now requires every district health authority to establish an LREC, the purpose of which being 'to consider the ethics of proposed research projects which will involve human subjects, and which will take place broadly within the NHS'. The LREC should consist of eight to twelve members, should include men and women from a wide age range, representatives of the nursing staff, hospital medical staff, general practitioners and at least two lay people. The posts of chair and vice-chair should be occupied by at least one of the lay members of the committee. The revised 1991 guidelines go a long way to remedy the inadequacies of earlier practices. LRECs should now be a standard size with a truly representative membership, and they must actually meet. Prior to 1991, some committees conducted their business entirely by post! But as we shall see when we look at the law and clinical research the LREC still lacks teeth.

Nursing research and LRECs

Proposals for nursing research within the NHS should also be submitted to an LREC. It may be argued that such research proposals should be reviewed by people with specialist knowledge of nursing rather than by a committee with a predominantly medical focus. Research carried out in nursing may use a variety of research methods, not all of which are invasive. If the emphasis is placed solely on protecting participants from physical harm as is often the case with purely medical research, then some nursing research may be considered to require less scrutiny than invasive research. Arguing in this way suggests that physical harm is of more importance than psychological or emotional harm. Although physical harm is easier to assess, it cannot be considered to be of greater importance. There is a danger of devaluing the nature and contribution of nursing research if it is perceived as being ethically unproblematic and not needing to go through more than a cursory review process. Nursing research should be subjected to ethical review to protect the well-being of patients and clients and to encourage nurses to undertake responsible research.

Changes in the NHS system resulting from the National Health Service and Community Care Act 1990 mean small district health authorities will soon be a thing of the past. Much larger health purchasing consortia will emerge from the amalgamation of local health authorities and such consortia will be far too large to manage with just one LREC. Either smaller regional-based committees will be called for or perhaps sub-committees should be discipline-based with an ethics committee expressly charged to review and monitor nursing research.

Research on vulnerable people

It may be argued that any person requiring the services of health professionals is vulnerable to exploitation and needs protection as a potential research subject. In many respects, this is what LRECs attempt to do when reviewing research proposals, but there are also certain groups of individuals who are particularly vulnerable as potential participants in research. Especially vulnerable groups include pregnant women, babies and children, the mentally ill, those who have learning difficulties, and unconscious patients. Vulnerable people may be less able to give informed consent, or they may be at high risk of developing side effects because of their special circumstances. Ideally research should not be carried out on such vulnerable groups at all and alternative research subjects should be found, but this may not be practical if the research study is specific to one of the identified groups. A new drug for pre-term infants must be proved to be safe and effective for pre-term infants.

Research committees reviewing research proposals using vulnerable people as potential research subjects have an onerous responsibility in judging whether such research is ethical. If the research subject cannot consent on his own behalf, cannot protect his own interests, then who should act for him? The 1991 Department of Health guidelines require consultation with next of kin. But the ultimate responsibility rests with the LREC in such cases. Research proposals can then be rejected if the participants are in danger of being harmed in some way. However, this does presuppose that the members of the ethical committee are impartial in their judgment and not influenced by the potential benefits of the research. This may be difficult to achieve if many of the members of the ethics committee are active researchers themselves as is often the case. The nurse can be seen as having a role as advocate for any participant in clinical research and especially for those patients and clients considered vulnerable. The UKCC in its document *Exercising Accountability* discusses the nurse's role in obtaining informed consent and the nurse would need to inform the researcher if she considered that the participant did not fully understand what was happening, or risked suffering significant harm or distress.

The law and research

Should you intend to carry out research on any animal, you are required by law to obtain a licence to do so from the Home Secretary under the Animals (Scientific Procedures) Act 1986. Home Office inspectors will judge whether the benefits likely from the proposed research justify the likely suffering entailed for the animal. If you plan an experiment on a human embryo *in vitro* of less than fourteen days' development, you must be licensed to carry out that experiment by the Human Fertilisation and Embryology Authority. As yet, as we have already noted, in the United Kingdom no legislation controls experimentation on born human beings. The justification advanced for providing statutory protection for animals and embryos, but not for you and me, is twofold. First, it is argued that the animal and the embryo have no choice: they are research conscripts. You can refuse to participate in research or prevent your child or vulnerable relative from being dragooned into a research trial. Second, the Department of Health maintains that the current informal system of regulating research via an LREC works very well.

There are three main legal issues, then, arising from research on human subjects.

1. Does the current system of regulation work to protect the legal interests of subjects?
2. Are the principles relating to consent satisfactory in the research context?
3. What provision is made to compensate an individual who suffers injury through involvement in research?

Ethical guidelines and the law

The ethical guidelines provided by codes such as the Nuremberg Code 1949 and the Declaration of Helsinki 1964 are not legally enforceable documents or rules. Their importance lies in the fact that the law requires that professionals attain the standard of a responsible body of professional opinion. If the general professional consensus is to adopt the ethical guidance as the standard then the law is likely to uphold and enforce that standard. Failure to comply with that standard with the result that a subject suffers injury may result in liability for negligence.

The Declaration of Helsinki itself does not offer full or detailed practical recommendations and so most EC states have introduced voluntary national guidelines. In addition to the Declaration of Helsinki, the United Kingdom has adopted a number of voluntary national guidelines including: ABPI (Association of British Pharmaceutical Companies) *Guidelines for Medical Experiments on Non-patient Human Volunteers* (1988) and *Clinical Trials Compensation Guidelines* (1991); Royal College of Physicians' *Guidelines on Research on Healthy Volunteers* (1990) and *Guidelines on the Practice of Ethics Committees in Medical Research involving Human Subjects* (1990); Department of Health guidelines on *Local Research Ethics Committees* (1991). These guidelines are supplementary to the Declaration but are still not comprehensive. Within the European Community a discussion paper has been prepared on the need for a Directive on Clinical Trials [III/3044/91(1991) January 23]. If the Directive is agreed, member states will have to pass specific legislation to regulate the conduct of trials or ensure that any existing legislation is in accordance with the Directive. So it may be that the European Community will ultimately force the United Kingdom to enact legislation giving express statutory force to the current morass of guidelines from different bodies on the ethics of research. For the moment, if a case went to court, the court would have to sift through the several sets of documents to identify proper professional practice.

The law and research ethics committees

As there is at present no legislation controlling the actual process and operation of clinical trials on humans, responsibility for their regulation has, as we have seen, been entrusted in the UK to local research ethics committees. We must now fill in a little more detail on the actual operation of an LREC. Since 1975 the Department of Health has required that each district health authority 'appoint a properly constituted local research ethics committee, which meets regularly, to register, review and approve (or not approve) the research conducted by its staff or using premises and facilities . . . and research undertaken by general practitioners within its boundaries'. (This requirement is currently imposed by the Department of Health guidelines, *Local Research Ethics Committees* (1991).) The NHS local research ethics committee is formally a sub-committee of the health authority. Therefore the health authority and each individual member of the committee owe a duty of care to anyone who participates in research approved by the ethics committee. The authority and the members of the committee have a legal responsibility to do that job properly. Although no case has yet reached an English court, they could be liable for any malpractice on their part.

Ethics committees have in the past varied greatly in their numbers, practices and effectiveness. The revised guidelines issued by the Royal College of Physicians in 1989 and the Department of Health in 1991 were designed expressly to introduce greater uniformity of practice. The emphasis of the guidelines is on the proper constitution of the LREC. A committee 'should command technical competence and judgment' and 'accommodate respected lay opinion'. Amongst other things committees should meet regularly and not conduct business by mail or telephone! They should use specialist referees to advise on any aspect of a research proposal where the committee itself lacks sufficient expertise in the area concerned. When reviewing each research proposal submitted the ethics committee must consider the following:

1. The scientific merit of the proposal.
2. Whether the subject's health may benefit from, or be affected by, the research.
3. Hazards to the subject and facilities to deal with hazards.
4. The degree of discomfort and distress to the subject.
5. Whether the investigator is adequately qualified or experienced.
6. Any financial or other rewards to the authority, doctors, researchers or subjects.
7. The need to ensure an adequate consent has been obtained from the subject.
8. Whether an appropriate information sheet for the subjects has been prepared.

All very well in theory, you may say, but what can an LREC do if researchers fail to submit proposals for approval or ignore the advice given by the committee? An NHS employee who fails to seek approval could be disciplined by her employing authority despite the fact that no law is contravened. Good practice now demands ethical approval outside the NHS, unapproved research could constitute professional misconduct. The RCP guidelines state: 'All medical research involving human subjects should undergo ethical review before it commences, in accordance with the principle that investigators should not be the sole judge of whether their research raises significant ethical issues.'

Consent to participation in trials

The fundamental principle of the Helsinki Declaration is that every subject 'must be adequately informed of the aims, methods, anticipated benefits and potential hazards of the study and the discomfort it may entail . . . The doctor should . . . obtain the subject's freely given informed consent, preferably in writing.'

Yet where therapeutic research is concerned, the Declaration makes an exception to the absolute requirement of obtaining such consent. If the researcher thinks that it is necessary not to obtain consent, she must give detailed reasons to an independent scrutiny committee, i.e. the LREC.

How far does English law conform to the tenets of the Declaration? Remember, in general health care treatment all that is required for a valid consent is that the patient be informed in broad terms what is to be done and why. And a claim in negligence for inadequate advice on consent, for insufficient disclosure of the risks of treatment, is judged by what constitutes acceptable professional opinion on disclosure. In the context of research the rules are almost certainly rather different. We would argue that a total failure to tell the patient he has been enrolled in a research trial invalidates his consent altogether. He has no understanding of the true nature of what he agrees to. Moreover, if he does expressly agree to enter a trial he must be given full and adequate information. Although there are still no legal cases reported on consent and research in England, remember that in *Sidaway* the Law Lords denied that they were handing over to the doctors unfettered control of information to patients. Lord Bridge in *Sidaway* said that 'the judge might in certain circumstances come to the conclusion that the disclosure of a particular risk was so obviously necessary to an informed choice on the part of the patient that no reasonable prudent medical man would fail to make it'. It would seem that failure to disclose risks involved in research would fall into that category. If a person is not told of known or suspected dangers of a particular trial he cannot be said to have been given any real choice.

Moreover, as the ethical guidelines are quite stringent as to informed consent, it is presumed that responsible professional practice must in any case conform to the ethical standards laid down. The ethical guidelines require that patients and volunteers are given full and sufficient information. Inadequate disclosure may even fall short of the inadequate *Sidaway* test.

Children in medical research programmes

The problems surrounding consent of children generally have been discussed in Chapter Nine. The *Gillick* case enables the minor to consent to treatment if he or she is judged to be sufficiently mature and intelligent to understand and reach a decision about the treatment proposed. The Family Law Reform Act 1969 empowers minors over sixteen to consent to medical treatment. In the case of therapeutic research the legal principles are probably the same. A different approach, however, might be taken to non-therapeutic research. The Family Law Reform Act does not apply to non-therapeutic research, it relates only to treatment. The position is probably this. The older child who truly understands what is entailed in volunteering to take part in non-therapeutic research can give consent herself or himself. Common sense suggests a dual consent be sought from both the older child and the parents right up until the child is legally an adult at eighteen.

Where younger children are concerned, therapeutic research poses little difficulty. If parents agree to a novel procedure in the hope that it will benefit their child, that consent will authorise the actions in question. The important proviso is that the decision should be made in the best interests of the child. Non-therapeutic research, though, is of no immediate benefit to the child. So can a parent authorise non-therapeutic research on her child for the benefit of the wider community? After all, the law limits the parental capacity to authorise procedures on their children to those procedures judged to be in the individual child's 'best interests'. In 1964 the Medical Research Council advised that non-therapeutic research on children was probably unlawful, but professional opinion has now changed. The British Paediatric Association considers research is lawful if the risk of harm to the child is negligible and parents give a fully informed consent on the child's behalf. Lawyers argue that if you reformulate the 'best interests' test as 'not against the interests of the child', limited non-therapeutic research on children may be lawful where that research is absolutely essential.

Incompetent adults and research

Mentally ill, those with learning disabilities or unconscious patients pose even greater problems. Remember, once someone reaches eighteen, no other person can give a legally effective consent to treatment on his or her behalf. In relation to treatment of persons unable to consent for themselves the House of Lords in *F* v. *West Berkshire AHA* (1989) held that a health professional could provide treatment to such a person providing that treatment was in the best interests of the patient and conformed to responsible professional practice. That doctrine can be applied with little difficulty to therapeutic research. The professional hopes to further the interests of the patient by entering him in the trial. Non-therapeutic research does not in any sense forward the interests of the subject. Ethical guidance sanctions non-therapeutic research on incompetent adults if the family agrees the risk is negligible and the research offers substantial benefit to patients suffering from the same illness or disability as the subject. Where competent patients could be used, incompetent patients should never be involved. It is not at all clear whether English law would endorse this ethical guidance, although it emanates from the Department of Health.

Compensation for mishap

If the subject of a clinical trial suffers personal injury through participation in the trial the only compensation available at present is as follows:

1. to subjects who can prove negligence on the part of the operator of the trial;
2. on an *ex gratia* basis.

Claims for negligence in respect of a randomised controlled trial may arise in two different contexts. A subject in the control group may complain that he was denied an improved prospect of cure. Subjects from the experimental group may allege that unjustifiable risks were taken. Success is unlikely in either case. For the control group subject, as long as conventional treatment remained proper practice, there can be no successful claim in negligence. In the case of the experimental group, as long as the new procedure was carried out in accordance with a responsible body of professional opinion, and was a properly conducted piece of research, that action is also likely to fail.

However, in any trial if the research team itself was careless in choosing subjects on the basis of their medical history, or in the conduct of the trial or in monitoring the effects of the trial, that carelessness creates a possible remedy for the patient. Theoretically he may also have a remedy against the ethics committee which approved the trial if they negligently approved a dangerous trial and were in breach of their undoubted duty to protect the interests of patients and volunteers. Problems of course lie in proof of negligence – this is likely to be even more difficult in the case of novel procedures than standard procedures.

The pharmaceutical industry operates *ex gratia* compensation schemes. For example, the Association of British Pharmaceutical Companies (ABPI) operates a scheme whereby any healthy volunteer in a drug trial initiated by an ABPI member will receive compensation for any injury arising from that trial. The problem is that many drug trials performed in British hospitals concern drugs manufactured by foreign companies. The Royal College of Physicians advises research ethics committees that they should obtain from such companies a written agreement to provide for research subjects a minimum of the same protection as that offered by the ABPI. Should such compensation be automatic for all those who volunteer to participate in research which ultimately benefits the whole community?

Monitoring research programmes

There is one exception to the informal, non-statutory regulation of research. In relation to new drugs, the drug licensing system established by the

Medicines Act 1968 enforces a degree of legislative control on drug trials. Normally, though not uniformly, a company seeking to try out a new drug on human volunteers must first obtain a clinical trial certificate (CTC). The CTC will only be granted if the company demonstrates that prior research, including, where relevant, animal tests, proves harm to humans unlikely. A complex reporting system monitors trials in progress. But the drug licensing system only addresses the inherent hazard of the trial and leaves overall ethical control in the hands of the LREC.

In the future European Community law may impose express legislation on clinical trials. Do you think anything less is satisfactory?

12

Nursing the dying

The process of dying and death itself are highly emotive and challenging issues. The issues are complex and varied both in terms of ethics and law. Advances in medical technology have meant that not only do many of us live longer, but also patients may be kept alive when, in the past, they would have died naturally. Patients may be resuscitated if their heart stops; mechanical ventilators and life-support machines enable seriously ill and injured patients to continue to live. Care of terminal illnesses in general has improved and lives may be prolonged through treatments such as radiotherapy, drug therapy and chemotherapy. The fundamental ethical and legal question has been whether health professionals should always seek to treat patients with terminal illnesses and always seek to prolong life.

Prolonging life

There are inevitably circumstances when a decision has to be made either to discontinue treating someone, or not to implement treatment in the first place. There are numerous examples in clinical practice. Consider the plight of patients in the terminal stages of diseases such as motor neurone disease or cancer, or babies born with lethal abnormalities such as Edwards syndrome. The idea of allowing people to die without intervention has existed from antiquity, but decisions of this sort have become increasingly important with the improvement in methods of intensive and critical care. Even the Roman Catholic Church, which still adheres to a strict interpretation of sanctity of life, defends the right of a patient to die with dignity, but that church, in conjunction with English law, does not consider that it is permissible to carry out active euthanasia, that is, deliberately to kill a patient even if they are not expected to recover.

One argument goes as follows: 'Thou shalt not kill, but needs't not strive officiously to keep alive' (Arthur Hugh Clough). In other words, although killing a patient is morally unacceptable, if a person is terminally ill with cancer, then should he suffer a cardiac arrest it would not be necessary to resuscitate him. This is a misinterpretation of the rhyme and given this meaning it misses the irony of Clough's point. There may be situations when this would appear to be a reasonable approach, for instance, when subjecting a patient to dramatic and often painful interventions would clearly not be in that patient's interests. The difficulty lies in deciding which interventions are basic requirements and which are not. It is often a distinction between 'ordinary' and 'extra-ordinary' means. Major surgery which is unlikely to cure the underlying disease or mechanical ventilation for a person diagnosed as brain dead may be classed as 'extra-ordinary means'. Keeping a patient warm, comfortable and pain-free and preventing pressure sores, all of which are required to meet the fundamental needs of a person, would be 'ordinary means'. Those are the 'easy' cases. However, some procedures and treatments are not so easily classified such as naso-gastric feeding. Food is an essential and basic requirement for life, but when the means used for feeding are artificial and even painful, and the patient is unconscious, does it become an 'extra-ordinary' measure? This was a crucial question in the case of Tony Bland, the young victim of the Hillsborough disaster who lay in a persistent vegetative state until the court declared that naso-gastric feeding could lawfully be withdrawn. It was believed that Tony had no hope of recovery and that he would never regain consciousness as we know it. But there are many other situations where a patient may be on the brink of death, but with prompt and appropriate treatment, may be brought back to consciousness and even improved health.

Resuscitation

All nurses are taught how to recognise a cardiac arrest and how to perform cardiopulmonary resuscitation, and they are expected to be fully conversant with the resuscitation procedures of the particular clinical area in which they are working. Although effective, cardiopulmonary resuscitation is not always an appropriate treatment for every patient, and health professionals often have to make decisions about when it is appropriate to resuscitate a dying person and when the person should be allowed to die. Often these decisions are made without consulting the patient and without their consent (although relatives may be involved in the decision-making process).

Clearly there are patients, such as those who are unconscious, whom it is not possible to consult about resuscitation, but it has been shown that even when patients could be consulted, doctors choose not to do so in many cases. To make a decision to allow someone to die without obtaining his consent disregards patient autonomy. So what are the arguments for not including the patient in the decision-making process? It may be thought that raising the subject for discussion is insensitive, or that the patient will not have enough specialist knowledge to understand why the decision has been made, or that the patient may disagree with the decision. Without doubt the subject is sensitive, but failure to recognise this fact and approach the subject sympathetically, using language the patient can understand, suggests poor communication skills. It is these skills which need refining. Health professionals may believe that they should always act in accordance with the principle of beneficence, but in doing so there is a real danger of being paternalistic. Patients who are capable of being consulted have both a legal and a moral right to exercise their own autonomy (see Chapter Four).

Nurses themselves are frequently excluded from the decision-making process despite the fact that, in many cases, it is the nurse who knows the patient and who will implement the emergency resuscitation procedure. It may be argued, according to the *Code of Professional Conduct*, that even if nurses are included in the decision-making process, they should abstain if the patient is excluded. Nurses are encouraged to 'work in an open and co-operative manner with patients, clients and their families, foster independence and recognise and respect their involvement in the planning and delivery of care' (clause five). However the Code also states that a nurse must 'work in a collaborative and co-operative manner with health care professionals and others involved in providing care, and recognise and respect their particular contributions within the care team' (clause six). This could be interpreted to mean that the nurse must either resuscitate or not resuscitate the patient according to the decision the doctor has made. While there are inequalities in the degree of participation in the decision-making process, the problem of conflicting roles will continue. The fact that the doctor has ultimate responsibility for the fate of the patient in hospital does not necessarily mean that the decision should be taken by the doctor alone. All those involved in the care of the patient should be consulted, but including nurses while excluding the competent patient from the decision-making process is not a better option than the exclusively medical model of decision-making and may be considered a form of non-voluntary euthanasia.

Euthanasia

The term euthanasia literally means 'good death' and one assumes that, given a choice free of legal and moral implications, the dying or suffering patient would choose the easiest and most pain-free release. Yet a patient may firmly believe in the sanctity of human life and that at all costs, and whatever the pain, he may not make a decision which would end his life and/or his suffering prematurely. So far as the patient is concerned, it is a matter of personal belief and choice. However, death, more so than any other physical or medical process, creates immense emotional, ethical and legal dilemmas, not so much for the patient, but rather for those who care for the dying. Perhaps it is the mystery of death itself and life thereafter which stirs the conscience. What do you do when your elderly aunt asks you to give her an overdose of sleeping pills because she has neither the strength to obtain them nor the energy to take them herself? Compassion, empathy, morality and conscience are all weighed against each other and then, of course, the consequences of your actions have to be considered, no doubt adding to the confusion. For the nurse, the ethical and legal debate surrounding euthanasia is of growing importance. As more and more terminally ill patients are cared for in the community, the likes of the Macmillan nurses and health visitors will be coping, often alone, with the difficulties of caring for the dying.

Yet what does a 'good death' mean? What are the patient's choices, if any, and how may they be effected? Euthanasia itself is a term which has a number of qualified meanings and it is only if these distinct meanings are understood that there can be an appreciation of the ethical and legal arguments and dilemmas. The primary distinction made is between active and passive euthanasia. Active euthanasia occurs when deliberate measures are taken to end a person's life, for example, by giving a lethal dose of a drug or poison. On the other hand, passive euthanasia involves the with-holding of treatment or life-saving measures from a dying person. A common example might be withholding antibiotics needed to cure a chest infection, which is likely to hasten the death of the patient already in the terminal stages of a disease.

Further distinctions are made within these two main categories. When the patient asks to be killed that is known as voluntary euthanasia. When a person is killed without their consent because they are incapable of being consulted, for example, a baby, this may be described as an act of involuntary euthanasia. Non-voluntary euthanasia defines the situation where a person is killed without his consent although he could have been consulted.

In law and in ethics distinctions have traditionally been made between active euthanasia and passive euthanasia. This debate is sometimes referred to as the distinction between positive acts which cause death, and omissions to act when action could have prevented death, i.e. letting the patient die. Philosophers such as Rachels and Singer in *Practical Ethics* have argued that there is no moral distinction between the two. But the law is clear in its support for the distinction however contradictory it may seem.

Acts and omissions

Active euthanasia, whether voluntary, involuntary or non-voluntary remains illegal in the UK, however humane the intention. Passive euthanasia, in certain circumstances, may be permissible. The following examples illustrate the difference (if there is one) between acts and omissions. A ninety-year-old patient has terminal cancer, is in great pain and asks to be helped to die. If the patient is given a lethal dose of potassium chloride, he will die quickly and an act of active euthanasia will have been carried out, hastening death and ending his suffering. Another ninety-year-old patient with terminal cancer is also in great pain but has not asked to die. He develops pneumonia, which if left untreated will kill him before the cancer does. The pneumonia can be treated with antibiotics but as the patient is dying, a decision is made to withhold the antibiotic therapy so that his suffering will not be prolonged. This is allowing death by omission – passive euthanasia. The intention in both of these cases is the same: to bring about the death of the patient and to end his suffering. Yet many health professionals believe that while the method described in the former case is not morally acceptable that described in the second is. Yet if the intention is the same, why is passive euthanasia not only permissible, but considered good practice, and yet active euthanasia impermissible?

The distinction in law is well illustrated by two recent cases. In 1992 Dr Cox was convicted of attempted murder after giving a terminally ill woman, who begged to be helped to die, an injection of potassium chloride. Yet, in 1993, following a request from his parents, the House of Lords gave permission for artificial feeding to be withdrawn from Tony Bland.

Intention

One possible way of differentiating between the morality of active and passive euthanasia is to consider what is intended by the health professionals involved. Suppose you are late for work one day. Whilst speeding in an attempt to make up for lost time you knock down and kill a pedestrian crossing the road. Although you have killed the person, you may argue that you did not intend to do so. Rather, your intention was to get to work as quickly as possible. On another day you are driving along at normal speed and you see someone you dislike. You accelerate, knock down and kill the person. Not only are you responsible for killing the person but you also intended to kill or at least injure them. Are situations in clinical practice analogous to this, for example, the practice of administering large doses of analgesia to terminally ill patients?

Consider the case of Mary who is terminally ill with cancer and in great pain. Dr White prescribes large doses of a drug, the side effects of which he knows will at least contribute to the cause of death. Like driving the car in the first instance, Dr White may argue that his intention is not to kill Mary but to relieve her pain. Another patient, John, is also terminally ill with cancer and in great pain; however his doctor, Dr Green, decides that the only way to end John's suffering is to give him an injection of a lethal substance like potassium chloride. This situation is similar to deliberately knocking the pedestrian down – Dr Green's intention is clearly to kill John. Dr White's actions are not as obvious. It could be argued that he is also killing the patient even though it is not his primary intention. He is treating the pain of the cancer rather than the cancer itself. In both cases the ultimate cause of death would not be cancer, Mary would die of the side effects of the analgesia and John would die from potassium toxicity.

At some stage Dr White must have made a decision not to treat Mary's cancer, but to make her as comfortable as possible until she dies, even if in doing so it means that she is given potentially lethal doses of analgesia. It would be difficult to argue that the doctor had not made this decision prior to prescribing the analgesia – it is difficult to imagine any other clinical situation where it would be considered good practice to give a patient potentially lethal doses of a drug. Consequently, some philosophers would argue that Dr White's intention (whatever his motive) is to bring about Mary's death and so there can be no moral difference between the actions of the two doctors. If it can be shown that there is no moral difference between actively and passively causing death, then why should one practice be considered right and the other wrong? Perhaps the difference in approach lies more in personal beliefs and individual morality – the difference between theory and practice.

Ends and means

The difference between deliberately killing a patient and letting a patient die may depend upon the end that has been decided upon and the means that are used to bring about that end. If a decision has been made not to treat a terminally ill patient, it does not follow that any action bringing about that death will be acceptable. Suppose that you decide you want a holiday in Australia, so you work extra hours and give up smoking to save the money for the plane ticket. You may decide that this will take too long, so you organise an armed robbery to get the funds. The goal in both cases is the same – to buy a plane ticket to Australia – but the means that you employ in order to attain that goal are quite different. Working extra hours and saving money would be acceptable means whereas armed robbery would not, because certain types of behaviour are considered to be morally acceptable and others such as lying and killing are not.

Dr White may admit that a decision has indeed been made not to treat Mary's cancer thereby allowing her to die. However, he could argue that, in making the decision, he is not suggesting that any means can be employed to bring about her death. Although Mary may die from the side effects of the drugs, for Dr White, this is justifiable and acceptable because his main purpose is to alleviate her pain. For this reason administering a dose of potassium chloride, which has no pain-relieving qualities, is not justifiable.

The psychological argument

Many health professionals argue that there is a psychological difference between active and passive euthanasia, that giving a patient an injection that directly causes death simply feels very different to giving large doses of drugs in the hope of controlling pain.

Suppose you are walking along a country lane and you see someone pick and eat some berries which you know are poisonous. The person dies as a result, but you refuse to accept any blame because you did not actually give her the berries to eat. You may argue that there is a psychological difference between actually giving a person poisonous berries and not informing her that the berries are poisonous. Clearly if she picked and ate them you could not be accused of attempting to kill her, but it might be a fairly natural response for you to feel guilty about withholding the information. Nor is it inconceivable that you might be criticised for not making an attempt to alert her to the fact that the berries were poisonous. Indeed, it is doubtful that you would be able to defend yourself to critics by arguing psychological differences.

Criticisms are often made against people who either turn a blind eye to events around them or who do not make rescue attempts when they could do so. For example, it has been argued that the German citizens who ignored what the Nazis were doing to the Jews were as guilty as those who actually carried out the murders, or that someone who does not attempt to rescue a person who has fallen overboard into the ocean is as guilty as if he had actually pushed the person. However, to hide Jews from the Nazis or to jump into the ocean to save another from drowning involves an element of personal risk. While it may be contended that individuals should feel an obligation to help others if in doing so they do not place themselves in any danger, this is not the same as imposing an obligation to be a hero.

Public confidence

Critics of active euthanasia also argue that such practices will undermine public confidence in the activities of health professionals. Patients will worry that decisions will be made to end their lives without being consulted or that other factors will be considered, such as economic pressures on health resources. The question is where or how will it all end. This is referred to as the 'slippery slope' or 'thin end of the wedge' argument. In the context of euthanasia the argument works like this. If euthanasia were allowed in certain specified circumstances, such as following a request from an incurably ill patient, we would have placed one foot on the slippery slope. Once on the slope it would be difficult to stop sliding down and might eventually result in accepting compulsory euthanasia. However, it is not always the case that once one sort of practice is accepted we are unable to distinguish between a clearly defined case and other more dubious practices. One example of this is noted by Rachels, who shows that while society tolerates killing in self-defence, allowing this practice has not resulted in the wholesale killing of innocent human beings.

Of course we do not know what sort of effect the introduction of legalised active euthanasia would have on society, but some argue that because of the possible negative consequences it is better not to take the risk. For example, it is known that the sooner organs are removed from the dying or dead donor, the better they are for transplantation. It has been argued that if people suspect the motives of health professionals in obtaining organs for transplantation, then permission may not be given for their removal. It could be that the focus of attention may shift from providing care which allows someone to die peacefully, to instigating aggressive treatment which favours the organ transplantation programme. The relationship between health professionals and patients is based on trust and this is essential for achieving high standards of patient care. Consequently it could be argued that if there is a possible threat to this relationship in allowing active euthanasia, the practice ought not to be allowed.

The euthanasia debate today

To many philosophers it seems illogical to condemn active euthanasia whilst condoning passive euthanasia. After all, the same end is to be achieved whatever the method or primary intention. However, to others the method is all important, as is the primary intention. Many would feel that their consciences would not allow them to carry out or be a party to active euthanasia, and that they should certainly not be under an obligation to do so; yet their consciences would be clear if they sat with a relative while the patient refused treatment and passed through the last hours of his life. For the dying person the answer may seem obvious – sanctity of life is either firmly entrenched or cedes to the right of self-determination. If the patient decides he wants to end his suffering there is little or no debate. Yet moral dilemmas abound for those who are asked to help or to do the deed. Compassion and deep-felt sympathy for a dying relative or friend racked with pain may well drive some to 'mercy killing' and they may justify their actions through love or their individual morality. But there are a great many who feel compassion but, for whatever personal and/or ethical reasons, cannot bring themselves actively to end a life. Whether it is a psychological difference or a matter of intention, it feels different actually to do it rather than to stand by and watch or wait.

Two recent court cases have highlighted the emotional, ethical and legal issues that surround the euthanasia debate today: the case of Doctor Cox and the case of Tony Bland.

Doctor Cox in the dock

Lilian Boyes had suffered from rheumatoid arthritis for twenty years and had been cared for by Nigel Cox, a consultant in rheumatology, for thirteen years. In August 1991 Mrs Boyes refused all medication apart from analgesia, and asked Dr Cox to end her life. Dr Cox informed her that he was not permitted to do so.

Although Diamorphine was administered to Mrs Boyes she remained in excruciating pain. On 16 August 1991, Dr Cox administered 100mg Diamorphine and 30mg of Diazepam to Mrs Boyes, and he fully expected that she would not survive for more than half an hour to an hour. Dr Cox visited Mrs Boyes shortly afterwards, but found she was still suffering. He administered 10ml of undiluted potassium chloride and recorded this in her notes. Mrs Boyes died soon afterwards.

Roisin Hart, the ward sister, arrived for a late shift soon after that and a nurse who had been on duty on the ward when Dr Cox had administered the drug informed Sister Hart and showed her the notes. After some deliberation Sister Hart reported the incident to her senior nurse manager on 21 August 1991.

Dr Cox was accused and convicted of attempted murder on 19 September 1992. He could not be charged with murder as by the time police started the investigation of the case Mrs Boyes's body had been cremated and the cause of death could not be established. He received one year's suspended sentence, and although he was found guilty of professional misconduct by the General Medical Council he was reinstated as a consultant in rheumatology, having agreed to certain conditions of employment. The GMC imposed the minimum possible penalty.

Although Dr Cox carried out a criminal act for which he received punishment, no doubt he would argue that he was acting in the interests of Mrs Boyes. He had known Mrs Boyes and her circumstances and it is easy to imagine the dilemma of a doctor genuinely concerned for his patient but unable to alleviate her pain, however hard he tried. Is the law wrong in not allowing this option of active euthanasia? In considering the question it is significant that critics of Dr Cox questioned his methods of pain relief; modern methods of palliative care for the dying ensure that patients do receive adequate pain relief, and professional updating in this area was one of the conditions of re-employment imposed by Dr Cox's employing authority.

Sister Hart's position in this case is of particular interest to nurses. In defending her action, Sister Hart said that she had no choice other than to report the incident to her manager in accordance with the *Code of Professional Conduct*, in particular clauses two and eleven. But was she right? Clause one states: 'act always in such a manner as to promote and safeguard the interests and well-being of patients and clients'. Mrs Boyes had expressed a wish to die and was in excruciating pain, so could it be argued that Sister Hart, by reporting the incident, was not protecting Mrs Boyes's interests at all? Sister Hart faced an unenviable dilemma but in the end she felt forced to report the incident because it was a criminal act.

Sister Hart was the ward sister which meant she had certain responsibilities for which she would be held accountable. The incident was brought to her attention by a member of her ward team and so the responsibility to decide what action, if any, was to be taken rested with her. She could of course have chosen to say nothing, but would then have had to defend her reasons for doing so if the matter resurfaced at a later stage. She would also have to account for failing to report a criminal act and might even have had to defend potential allegations of misconduct herself.

Letting Tony Bland die

The Hillsborough football disaster in April 1989 was a national tragedy. Ninety-five people were killed and many others were seriously injured, but the tragedy did not end there. The plight of Tony Bland, who was crushed at the grounds, was followed and debated until his eventual death and thereafter.

After his initial injury Tony required mechanical ventilation for one week, but he was later able to breathe spontaneously. A diagnosis was ultimately made that Tony was in a persistent vegetative state. He would remain permanently and irreversibly unconscious. He had lost all capacity for any voluntary movement. He required twenty-four hour nursing care, was fed through a naso-gastric tube and any acquired infection was treated with antibiotics.

Following discussions with Tony's parents, the consultant caring for him sought advice from the coroner on the legal implications if a decision were made to remove Tony's feeding tube, or if antibiotic therapy were withheld. The coroner advised that under the current law in England and Wales, a person acting in such a way would be charged with murder. A request was made to the High Court in November 1992 to allow Tony's feeding tube to be removed, and a declaration was made that this action would be lawful. The decision was upheld by the House of Lords, the feeding tube was removed and Tony died soon afterwards.

Considered medical opinion was that Tony would never recover from being in a persistent vegetative state but if his current care were continued he would be likely to survive for many years. The House of Lords stated that, in general, it would not be lawful for a doctor to discontinue treatment of an unconscious patient, but that he was under no obligation to continue to treat a patient where there was no possible benefit to the patient.

Should the question of benefit include interests beyond those of the patient himself? Should Tony's parents' interests, their need to grieve, be taken into consideration? What about the emotional and physical pressures on the health professionals caring for him? These may well be valid and necessary factors, but in future will decisions like this include considerations of the costs of keeping a PVS patient alive? Finally we may also want to question whether long and protracted legal cases are the right way to solve dilemmas such as this and who should ultimately make the decision about discontinuing any sort of treatment. The *Bland* case attracted intense media coverage and individuals and groups opposed to the removal of Tony's feeding tube protested at the gates of the hospital caring for him. Equally vociferous were the supporters of the action. What is clear is that this test case will certainly have implications for future cases and that the ethical debate about the moral acceptability of such a practice will continue.

The law's approach to euthanasia

The nurse cannot only be concerned with the ethical debates on euthanasia. The law has as great an impact and is the ultimate judge of her conduct. For the lawyer the debate starts from a slightly different point from that of the philosopher. It is necessary to consider first what actually constitutes death for legal purposes. The whole nature of the ethical debate could change if the definition of death were different.

The definition of death

The law requires that there be a particular point at which death can be and is acknowledged. It is legally important for the purposes of succession and inheritance of property. A murder victim must die within one year and one day of the initial wrongful act if the accused is to be charged with murder. Probably the most persuasive reason for a definition of death or, at least, criteria against which death can be diagnosed is the ever-advancing transplantation programme so that organs can never be removed before a person is medically and legally dead.

Today death is defined in these complex situations as 'brain stem death'. Without a functioning brain stem, acceptable life is impossible. The brain stem is the part of the brain that controls vegetative functions including breathing. If 'brain stem death' is diagnosed, a person is medically and legally dead whether or not the function of other organs may be maintained by artificial means.

The definition is a medical definition and not a legal one. The main purpose of the procedure is to provide a scientific basis upon which a decision can be made that patients who will no longer benefit may be removed from ventilator or other life support. In light of this purpose and

the Tony Bland case it may well be that the current definition will have
to be redefined once again, in time, to include non-biological considerations such as the quality of life. Tony Bland was not dead according to
brain stem death criteria. None the less the House of Lords upheld a
declaration that naso-gastric feeding and antibiotic care could lawfully be
withheld and that therefore he be allowed to die. UK law imposes no
conditions as to how the diagnosis should be made. The law appears to
be happy to accept the decisions of medical practitioners, which enables
the law to adopt changes in medical approach without the need to amend
static definitions.

A statutory definition of death?

There is much debate as to whether there should be a statutory definition
of death. A statutory definition would provide certainty, but in any event
would have to be based on scientific opinion. Certainty is clearly an advantage but the ensuing disadvantage is that a legislative definition may
not be flexible enough to allow for changes in medical opinion or advances
in medical technology. If, on the other hand, a formula were devised which
allowed for such flexibility, there is the danger that it would not provide
sufficient safeguards against abuse and misapplication. The legislative process
takes time and may not always be able to respond speedily to urgent or
novel situations.

There are many factors which have to be examined when considering
a statutory formula. Take, for example, the switching off of life-support
machines. There are two distinct situations: first, where the machine is
turned off because it is medically established that the patient is dead; and
second, where the machine is switched off because there is no further
justification in continuing artificial life support and a decision is made to
allow the patient to die. In the second situation, a decision to discontinue
'extra-ordinary' treatment involves considerations such as consent, quality
of life, and the proper use of scarce resources. These issues do not arise
where the machine is turned off because the patient has been declared
dead. However, without proper safeguards, medical changes in the definition of death could allow in by the back door limited forms of euthanasia.
Such decisions should not be left to doctors and judges alone. However,
great care would have to be taken in devising a formula and the task is
certainly not an easy one. The main concern must be that at least some
safeguards should be put in place in order that the debate is taken outside
the exclusively medical and judicial arenas.

Law and the euthanasia debate

Defining death is only part of the problem. The euthanasia debate involves
a huge number of ethical questions which have only very recently begun

to be discussed in the United Kingdom legal forum. It really was not until the highly publicised trial of Dr Cox that judicial consideration of the euthanasia debate became unavoidable in the United Kingdom.

In the context of euthanasia especially, law and ethics are inseparable. Does the patient have a right protected by law to human dignity and to die with dignity? Answers to such questions are both necessary and desirable, especially for patients sustained on life-support machines, incurable unconscious patients who must be artificially fed or ventilated, and those who are conscious but terminally ill.

The approach of the law has been timid mainly because of the controversy and emotion involved and because of the fear of where it all might lead. What is clear is that the law retains the distinction between active and passive euthanasia, however many moral philosophers may dislike it. Until Parliament chooses to act, this will remain the common law position on ending life. The principle is as follows:

> the law draws a crucial distinction between cases in which a doctor decides not to provide, or to continue to provide, for his patient treatment or care which could or might prolong his life, and those in which he decides, for example by administering a lethal drug, actively to bring his patient's life to an end. . . . the former may be lawful, either because the doctor is giving effect to his patient's wishes by withholding the treatment or care, or even in certain circumstances in which . . . the patient is incapacitated from stating whether or not he gives his consent. But it is not lawful for a doctor to administer a drug to his patient to bring about his death, even though that course is prompted by a humanitarian desire to end his suffering, however great that suffering may be. . . . So to act is to cross the Rubicon which runs between on the one hand the care of the living patient and on the other hand euthanasia – actively causing his death to avoid or end suffering. Euthanasia is not lawful at common law. (Lord Goff, *Airedale NHS Trust* v. *Bland* 1993, p. 867)

It is upon this fundamental distinction in the care of the dying that the following discussion on nursing the dying is based. It is important in every situation which presents ethical and legal health care problems that emphasis be placed on the whole team of professionals. It is especially important in the euthanasia debate when the effects of treatment decisions will inevitably fall on nursing staff who will care for the dying person whether it be in hospital or in the community.

Murder: active voluntary or involuntary euthanasia

Murder is the deliberate taking of another person's life, whether or not that person is dying. Causing the death of another by a reckless or grossly negligent act, without any intention to kill, can constitute the crime of manslaughter, for example, reckless driving or gross negligence in the care of a patient which results in death. It has always been clear that to act positively to hasten death or end the life of another is murder. The criminal law distinguishes between doing a positive act which causes death and omitting to do an act which would have prevented death. Usually an omission to prevent death will not give rise to a conviction for murder or manslaughter unless it can be shown that the accused was under a duty to the deceased to do what he omitted to do. For the nurse, then, the relevant question relates to the extent of the duty owed to the dying person.

Where the intention is to kill a fit and healthy person the law will not hesitate to prosecute and convict the killer if guilt is proved beyond reasonable doubt. With 'mercy killing' the intention is still to kill but the motive is generally kind. There is no doubt that as 'mercy killing' is illegal, motive is largely irrelevant, but there are ways in which the law has shown lenience to relatives who seek to end their loved one's suffering. It has not been unknown for the Director of Public Prosecutions to refuse to prosecute a 'mercy killer' despite clear evidence. Even where prosecutions are initiated, the courts may choose to deal with the accused compassionately. Lenience is possible if the charge is that of manslaughter where the judge has discretion in sentencing; murder on the other hand carries a mandatory sentence of life imprisonment. Clearly any nurse who practised active euthanasia, regardless of compassion, would open himself to charges of murder, attempted murder or manslaughter if the facts could be established.

There is one notable exception to the absolute ban on deliberate killing, laid down by Mr Justice Devlin in the case of *R* v. *Adams* (1957). Dr Adams was charged with the murder of an eighty-one-year-old patient who had suffered a stroke. It was alleged that he had prescribed and administered such large quantities of heroin and morphine, that he must have known that the drugs would kill her. The judge restated the law that health care practitioners were in no special or separate category and were subject to the law of murder if they end the life of a dying patient. He went on to say:

> but that does not mean that a doctor who was aiding the sick and dying had to calculate in minutes, or even hours, perhaps not in days or weeks, the effect on a patient's life of the medicines which he would administer. If the first purpose of medicine – the restoration of health – could no longer be achieved, there was still much for the doctor to do and he was entitled to do all that was proper and necessary to relieve pain and suffering even if the measures he took might incidentally shorten life by hours or perhaps even longer. The doctor who decided whether or not to administer the drug could not do his job if he were thinking in terms of hours or months of life. Dr Adams's defence was that the treatment was designed to promote comfort, and if it was

the right and proper treatment, the fact that it shortened life did not convict
him of murder. (p. 375)

This is otherwise known as the principle of 'double effect'. That is to say,
if an act has two inevitable consequences, one good and one bad, the act
may be justified in certain circumstances. Mr Justice Devlin's statement has
been widely accepted as representing the law on the issue of treatment of
terminally ill patients. In alleviating pain it is legally permissible to ignore
the fact that the treatment involved may hasten the patient's death. If,
however, it can be shown that the administration of the drug was designed
to kill the patient and not to alleviate pain or improve comfort, that would
be a case of murder or attempted murder as it was in the *Cox* case.

The *Cox* case offers no new legal guidelines in relation to the euthanasia
debate. The *Adams* case still stands as authority for the legal force of the
principle of double effect. Had Dr Cox administered a drug which pos-
sessed at least some analgesic qualities he would almost certainly not have
been prosecuted and sentenced. The reality of the situation is that had
Roisin Hart not informed the hospital authorities, Dr Cox might not have
been found out. Mrs Hart's delay in reporting Lilian Boyes's death meant
that the autopsy could not prove beyond doubt that the injection was the
actual cause of death. This enabled Mr Justice Ognall to consider Dr Cox's
case under the charge of attempted murder rather than murder. Had Dr
Cox been charged and convicted of murder the judge would have had to
sentence him to life imprisonment.

The case highlights the important role of nurses in all health care decisions. It is only fairly recently that judicial acknowledgement of team work
and joint responsibility for decision-making has been made. Undoubtedly
Dr Cox faced an extreme problem in treating Lilian Boyes when huge
doses of Diamorphine failed to relieve her pain. Roisin Hart faced a professional and ethical dilemma. Her actions, whatever her motives and
intentions, were legally significant. It is clear that mercy killing is murder
unless the principle of double effect can be invoked. Potassium chloride
has no pain-relieving qualities. Yet if Mrs Hart had not reported this
action the issue would not have been brought to the attention of the public
and the courts. Whatever your moral views on euthanasia, the minimum
standard that should be set, if it is to be allowed in any form, is that a
decision to end life should never be made by only one person. Dr Cox, it
is reported, had spoken with Mrs Boyes and her family and two other
consultants. However, he also shared responsibility for her care with other
medical and nursing staff and they too, it is argued, should have been
consulted. If such unilateral decisions are made, then the result will be that
doctors alone, without any safeguards, would be practising active and
passive euthanasia. Without safeguards such power could be open to abuse.
At least if a majority team decision is made, there are some safeguards.

Assisting suicide

The criminal law is also important in the context of the relationship between suicide and the euthanasia debate. It could be argued that supplying tablets to enable a patient to take an overdose or switching off a life-support machine both amount to assisting or aiding and abetting suicide. Under the Suicide Act 1961 it is no longer a criminal offence to commit, or attempt to commit, suicide but 'a person who aids, abets, counsels or procures the suicide of another or an attempt by another to commit suicide, shall be liable on conviction . . . to a term not exceeding fourteen years'. In relation to health care workers it would in practice be very difficult to prove that a doctor or nurse who had supplied drugs to a patient was responsible for the patient taking an overdose and at common law the refusal of life-sustaining treatment is not a matter of attempted suicide. It is recognised as a matter of self-determination as was made clear in the *Bland* judgment. If, however, a nurse counselled a patient on methods of suicide, intending the patient to commit suicide as a result of the counselling, this could be an offence under the Act.

But what of the many situations in which the patient will be unable to take his own life or simply may not want to do so himself? In these situations what is the alternative when the patient no longer wants to live?

Is there a 'right' to refuse treatment and to die?

Does a right to self-determination encompass a legal right to insist that medical treatment be withdrawn so that the patient be permitted to die? The answer is complicated and may depend on the type of situation involved. A competent adult patient might decide, while coping with an incurable disabling disease or terminal illness, that he would rather die. The first option is suicide. This, however, may not be a viable option for some patients. A patient may be conscious but maintained on a respirator, perhaps in the terminal stage of motor neurone disease. Others are fully conscious but incapacitated so that they breathe naturally but must be fed and cared for, such as paraplegics and tetraplegics. Patients do have a basic right to self-determination: in the first place they do not have to seek medical advice and treatment; and any touching or interference without consent normally constitutes trespass. A patient may discharge himself from medical care and thereby any further unconsented treatment will also constitute a trespass. On strict logical reasoning, the wishes of a competent patient, or of a formerly competent patient who had made his wishes known while competent, should be respected. The question is whether that logic is fully recognised by the law.

Inroads have been made regarding legal concepts of self-determination and consent (see Chapter Four). But self-determination is a fundamental principle. In *Bland* Lord Goff stated:

> it is established that the principle of self-determination requires that respect must be given to the wishes of the patient, so that if an adult patient of sound mind refuses, however unreasonably, to consent to treatment or care by which his life would or might be prolonged, the doctors responsible for his care must give effect to his wishes, even though they do not consider it to be in his best interests to do so. . . . To this extent, the principle of sanctity of human life must yield to the principle of self-determination. . . . On this basis, it has been held that a patient of sound mind may, if properly informed, require that life support should be discontinued. (p. 866)

However, in practice, patients' wishes have often been overridden and treatment has been given. There are medical arguments to suggest that in life-threatening situations patients are not always capable of making rational decisions – they may no longer be 'competent'. Will the law protect doctors and nurses who save or prolong the lives of patients against their wishes? If carers do impose treatment may they find themselves liable for battery as in *Malette* v. *Shulman* (1988) (Ontario High Court)?

The answer would appear to be this. If it is clear beyond doubt that a patient, voluntarily and fully understanding the implications of his decision, rejects further treatment, then any act directly contravening his wishes to cease treatment will be unlawful. When there is some real doubt about the patient's understanding or the voluntariness of his refusal of treatment the court may in turn be prepared to give the health professional the benefit of the doubt (*Re T* (1992)).

But there is a further worry for a nurse involved in a decision to withdraw life support, for example by switching off a ventilator or removing a naso-gastric tube. Regardless of the patient's wishes, is the nurse participating in an act that hastens death? Does he risk being charged with murder? As we noted earlier, it is no defence to a charge of murder that the patient asked to be killed. The House of Lords in *Bland* appear to have decided that withdrawal of life support should not be treated any differently from withholding fresh treatment. Switching off a ventilator or withdrawing a feeding tube is thus simply classified as an omission to continue treatment. There is no criminal liability for omissions unless there is a duty to act. The outcome depends now on the legal duty owed by a health care professional to a patient in such a situation. If the patient refuses further treatment which has proved to be ineffective, the health professional is under no duty to continue treatment and this is so whether or not the patient is competent. Selective non-treatment has gained acceptance as part of good medical practice and it is acceptable to confine treatment to 'ordinary measures' being defined according to personal circumstances, the law, the times and the culture. Other factors too may be relevant such as the underlying condition, the physical and psychological pain of treatment, claims on scarce resources and general prospects for patient and family.

The unconscious patient

The conscious patient's request that further life support be terminated concerns problems of distinguishing between medical acts and omissions. The difficulties are yet more complex where the patient has been rendered unconscious by illness or injury and is unlikely ever to regain consciousness. In the United Kingdom, unlike many American states, there is no constitutional right of privacy and, as yet, no legally enforceable doctrine of substituted judgment, whereby a proxy known to the patient is appointed to make a decision based on what he thinks the patient would have decided.

Some of the issues surrounding unconscious patients were addressed by the House of Lords in the *Bland* case. The Official Solicitor acting on behalf of Tony argued that doctors and nursing staff had a continuing duty to feed Tony by naso-gastric tube and that if they terminated such life-sustaining treatment they would be guilty of manslaughter. He tried to argue that naso-gastric feeding was indistinguishable from normal feeding – simply an ordinary measure. The House of Lords held that Tony's carers would not be acting unlawfully if they discontinued artificial feeding which was described by the House as an 'invasive medical procedure'.

Lord Keith stated that if continued treatment would benefit an unconscious patient in some way it would not be lawful for a carer simply to stop treatment. In this case, however, it was decided that there was no duty to continue treatment, where a large body of informed and responsible medical opinion maintained that no benefit would be conferred on the patient.

The House of Lords was careful to avoid establishing a precedent for passive euthanasia on any large scale in the *Bland* case. Clear attempts were made to set limits on the remit of the case and the House emphasised that they were not seeking to develop new law in the area of euthanasia. The decision was specific to the facts of the case itself. *Bland* is important in that it provides justification for a limited form of passive euthanasia in a way which largely removes responsibility for the death from those who ultimately withhold treatment. Their Lordships directed their attention towards the duty owed by health carers to the dying patient. The key to the judicial reasoning lies in the formulation of the question 'whether artificial feeding and antibiotic drugs may lawfully be withheld from an insensate patient with no hope of recovery when it is known that if that is done the patient will shortly thereafter die' (Lord Goff, p. 865). In determining that issue the question to be asked is 'not whether it is in the

best interests of the patient that he should die. The question is whether it
is in the best interests of the patient that his life should be prolonged by
the continuance of this form of medical treatment or care' (p. 869).

The Law Lords decided that even though the intention was to bring
about Tony's death there would be no criminal act because it was not in
his interests to continue the life-supporting care and treatment. The doctors responsible for Tony's care had come to the conclusion that it would
be to his benefit to withdraw life support. That conclusion was in accordance with the proposals contained in the Discussion Paper on *Treatment
of Patients in Persistent Vegetative State* issued by the BMA Medical Ethics Committee in 1992. In this way the *Bolam* test requiring that a practice
accord with a responsible body of professional opinion was satisfied and
on that basis, the House of Lords decided the treatment could lawfully be
withheld. Hence the carers would not be guilty of murder when they
discontinued treatment and they would not be civilly liable. The justification for discontinuation lay in the futility of the treatment.

According to Lord Keith it is simply that there is no duty to continue
treatment if no benefit will be conferred. Existence in a permanent vegetative
state cannot be considered to be a benefit and therefore this fact provided
a proper basis for the decision to discontinue treatment. Lord Goff supported the argument that discontinuing life support should be classified as
an omission to act. The duty owed to the patient was to decide whether
it was in his best interests to continue life-prolonging treatment. The doctor's
duty is not one of continuing treatment at all costs. Indeed, continuing to
impose treatment which contravened the patient's interests might itself be
unlawful. If there was no justification for maintaining the violation of
Tony Bland's body, dignity and privacy, in terms of benefit to him, that
violation itself could be seen as a continuing battery against his insensate
person. The nurse caring for a patient in a persistent vegetative state can
play a full role in assessing the interests of the patient and participating in
the judgment as to when the time has come for treatment to cease.

But the *Bland* judgment, while largely deferring to the opinion of health
professionals to determine when continuing treatment cannot possibly confer
any benefit on the patient, does not hand powers of life and death over to
those professionals. The House of Lords ruled that in any subsequent case
where health professionals judged that artificial feeding or ventilation should
be discontinued in a patient who was not 'brain stem' dead, an application
should be made to the court for a declaration on the legality of what is
proposed. Their lordships appeared to limit the freedom to act as Tony
Bland's doctors did to cases where, after full investigation of the facts, the
unfortunate patient was established to be without doubt in a permanent
vegetative state and all were agreed that he could never regain any level
of meaningful human existence. Yet just a year after *Bland* in *Frenchay
Healthcare NHS Trust* v. *S* (1994) the Court of Appeal appeared to say

that as long as there was sufficient responsible medical evidence in support of discontinuing feeding, the courts would in effect 'rubber stamp' the doctors' decisions. Should doctors (or nurses) have such power?

Advance directives

If someone does not want others to decide his fate when he can no longer speak for himself he may consider drawing up an advance directive. Advance directives are documents which set out in advance of incompetence, through ageing, accident or disease, how a person wishes to be treated. There are two forms of advance directives.

1. A 'living will' may be executed whereby the person declares the circumstances in which those caring for him should cease any life-sustaining treatment. A 'living will' may provide, amongst other things, that if he develops terminal cancer, but is no longer competent, he should not be given antibiotics to fight any life-threatening infection, and should not be artificially fed.
2. He may execute a 'durable power of health care attorney', whereby he nominates a proxy to act on his behalf and make treatment decisions for him should he become incompetent.

Usually 'living wills' and 'durable powers of attorney' will be complementary. The patient will use the 'living will' to indicate his general wishes, and then nominate a proxy to apply the 'will'.

There is nothing to stop any English patient from executing a 'living will'. As yet their legality has not been fully tested in the English courts. It is, however, thought that such documents would be recognised by the courts and could be enforced on practitioners. Such optimism derives from the case of *Re T* where the patient had signed a form of refusal to a blood transfusion and the court was asked to decide upon its validity. In order for any such refusal of consent to be binding, the Court of Appeal decided that four criteria had to be fulfilled as follows:

1. The patient must have capacity to make the decision (i.e. must not be mentally ill and must be free from the influence of drugs).
2. The patient must not have been unduly influenced by a third party.
3. The patient must have understood in broad terms the nature and effect of the treatment which is being refused.
4. The refusal must cover the actual situation in which treatment is needed.

On the actual facts of *Re T* (see Chapter Four) those criteria were found not to be established. However, that judgment expressly recognised the patient's right to state in advance, and in writing, his or her objection to certain forms of treatment. By analogy it would seem that such recognition could be stretched at least to 'living wills'. For a durable power of health care attorney to have legal force, legislation would have to be enacted because there is no legal authority at present which allows one person to act as a proxy on behalf of another adult patient. But the Law Commission has recently made a proposal in favour of legal recognition of durable powers of attorney (Law Commission Consultation Paper No. 129).

The greatest problem with 'living wills' and durable powers of health care attorney is that any sort of advance directive can only authorise an act which the patient, if competent, can authorise. It may authorise cessation of treatment, within limits as previously discussed, but cannot, however, authorise any act of active euthanasia. The 'living will' may well prevent the doctors administering antibiotics when the patient contracts pneumonia in the terminal stage of dying from cancer. It cannot authorise the doctor to end the patient's pain with a swift, lethal injection.

Legislation?

The English law surrounding euthanasia, despite the *Cox* and *Bland* cases, offers little by way of certainty or logic. Lilian Boyes who wanted to die had no right to be helped to do so. Tony Bland who felt nothing could be 'starved' to death. If Dr Cox had used a different drug to end Mrs Boyes's suffering he might never have faced trial. The professionals and family caring for any other patient like Tony Bland in a persistent vegetative state will also have to run the gauntlet of the courts and the press.

This chaotic state of affairs has led to calls for legislative reform. But when the ethical and moral issues are so diverse, how do you legislate on dying a 'good death'? There are two possible ways in which legislative reform could take shape. The first is to introduce legislation which provides for, much more clearly than at present, the circumstances in which health professionals must cease to continue attempts to prolong life. So, for example, the legislation would provide for cases like Tony Bland, where a medical decision has been made that there is no further benefit for the patient in continuing treatment. In doing so the legislation could, at the same time, give binding force to advance directives and clarify the procedure by which these decisions are made. Such reform would necessarily require consideration and a formulation of the extent to which the families of terminally ill or comatose patients should be involved in the process. The second, and more radical approach, is to enact legislation which permits active euthanasia in certain circumstances. Without doubt this would incite much vitriolic debate simply in defining the permitted circumstances, not to mention fierce opposition from pro-life groups and those who adhere to the doctrine of sanctity of life. There will also be enormous practical difficulties in drafting such legislation. Would the result be death on demand, not only from the dying individual, but from relatives and other 'interested' parties? How would individuals be safeguarded from exploitation? These questions and concerns have already been raised in observing countries in which active euthanasia is currently permitted. In the Netherlands doctors are not prosecuted for assisting patients to die as long as certain guidelines laid down by the medical association are met. But opponents of euthanasia express concern that the theoretical limits are vague. There are suggestions that non-voluntary and involuntary euthanasia are practised and the extent to which euthanasia is in reality practised is uncertain. How slippery is the slope? Any attempt at legislation must take all of these factors, and more, into account.

Conclusion

There is clear demand for Parliamentary and public debate on the issue of euthanasia. The judges are unhappy about making decisions where there is so little firm legal guidance and patients continue to suffer amidst the confusion and ambiguity. The Law Commission is considering the status of advance directives, and most recently the House of Lords Select Committee on Medical Ethics held a wide-ranging review of the law relating to care of the dying. The Committee's Report endorsed the use of 'living wills' and recognised that heroic treatment to prolong the process of dying was ill-judged. The wishes of the patient should be paramount when decisions have to be made about continuing treatment. However, the Committee came out firmly opposed to any reform of the law to decriminalise any form of active euthanasia. The difficulties entailed in such a radical reform were perceived as insurmountable.

Sources and further reading

ABPI (Association of British Pharmaceutical Companies) (1988), *Guidelines for Medical Experiments in Non-Patient Volunteers*, London.

ABPI (1991), *Clinical Trials Compensation Guidelines*, London.

Bainham, A. (1992), The judge and the competent minor, *Law Quarterly Review*, 108, pp. 194–200.

Beauchamp, T. L., and J. F. Childress (1989), *Principles of Biomedical Ethics*, 3rd ed., Oxford, Oxford University Press.

Bok, S. (1982), *Secrets*, Oxford, Oxford University Press.

Brazier, M. (1990), Sterilisation: down the slippery slope?, *Professional Negligence*, VI, pp. 25–7.

Brazier, M. (1992), *Medicine, Patients and the Law*, Harmondsworth, Penguin, Chapters 3–7, 11, 13–15, 19.

Bridgeman, J. (1993), Old enough to know best?, *Legal Studies*, 13, pp. 69–80.

British Medical Association (1993), *Treatment of Patients in Persistent Vegetative State*, London, BMA.

Brykczynska, G. M. (ed.) (1989), *Ethics in Paediatric Nursing*, London, Chapman Hall.

Clough, A. H., 'The latest decalogue', in Glover, J. (1977), *Causing death and saving lives*, Harmondsworth, Penguin, p. 92.

Cormack, D. F. S. (ed.) (1991), *The Research Process in Nursing*, 2nd ed., Oxford, Blackwell.

Cram, I. (1990), Access to health records, *New Law Journal*, 140, p. 1382.

Department of Health (1991), *Local Research Ethics Committees* (HSG (91) 5), Heywood, DOH.

Douglas, G. (1991), *Law, Fertility and Reproduction*, London, Sweet and Maxwell, Chapter 3, pp. 27–39, Chapter 5, pp. 73–102, Chapter 8, pp. 169–98.

Duff, R. F. and A. G. M. Campbell (1973), Moral and ethical dilemmas in the special care nursery, *New England Journal of Medicine*, 289, pp. 890–4.

Dworkin, R. (1977), *Taking Rights Seriously*, London, Duckworth.

Finch, J. (1982), Paternalism and professionalism in childbirth – I and II, *New Law Journal*, 132, pp. 995–6 and 1011–12.

Gillon, R. (1985), *Philosophical Medical Ethics*, Chichester, Wiley.

Glover, J. (1977), *Causing Death and Saving Lives*, Harmondsworth, Penguin.

Greenwalt, K. (1987), *Conflicts of Law and Morality*, New York, Oxford University Press.

Harris, J. (1985), *The Value of Life*, London, Routledge.

Harris, J. (1986), The survival lottery, in P. Singer (ed.), *Applied Ethics*, Oxford, Oxford University Press.

Hart, H. L. A. (1968), *Punishment and Responsibility*, Oxford, Oxford University Press.

Hoggett, B. (1988), The royal prerogative in relation to the mentally disordered: resurrection, resuscitation, or rejection, in M. D. A. Freeman (ed.), *Medicine, Ethics and the Law*, London, Stevens.

Hoggett, B. M. (1990), *Mental Health Law*, 3rd ed., London, Sweet and Maxwell.

Houghton-James, H. (1992), The child's right to die, *Family Law*, 22, pp. 550–4.

House of Lords Select Committee on Medical Ethics (1994), *Report*, London, HMSO.

Jones, M. (1989), Justifying medical treatment without consent, *Professional Negligence*, V, pp. 178–84.

Jones, M. (1990), Medical confidentiality and the public interest, *Professional Negligence*, VI, p. 16.

Kennedy, I. (1976), The legal effect of requests by the terminally ill and aged not to receive further treatment from doctors, *Criminal Law Review*, pp. 217–32.

Kennedy, I. (1977), Switching off life support machines: the legal implications, *Criminal Law Review*, pp. 443–52.

Kennedy, I. and A. Grubb (1994), *Medical Law*, London, Butterworths.

Keown, J. (1992), The law and practice of euthanasia in the Netherlands, *The Law Quarterly Review*, 108, pp. 51–78.

Khuse, H. and P. Singer (1985), *Should the Baby Live?*, Oxford, Oxford University Press.

Kings College (1992), *Manual for Research Ethics Committees*, London, Kings College.

Korgaonkar, G. and D. Tribe (1992), Living wills: their legal status, *Solicitors Journal*, 136, p. 960.

Law Commission Paper No. 129 (1993), Mentally incapacitated adults and decision-making, London, HMSO.

Lee, S. (1986), *Law and Morals: Warnock, Gillick and Beyond*, London, Oxford University Press, Chapters 1, 6, 14.

Lockwood, M. (1985), When does life begin?, in M. Lockwood (ed.), *Moral Dilemmas in Modern Medicine*, Oxford, Oxford University Press.

MacDonald, M. (1984), Natural rights, in J. Waldron (ed.), *Theories of Rights*, Oxford, Oxford University Press.

McHale, J. (1992), Whistleblowing in the NHS, *Journal of Social Welfare and Family Law*, V, p. 363.

McHale, J. (1993), Whistleblowing in the NHS revisited, *Journal of Social Welfare and Family Law*, I, p. 52.

MacIntyre, A. (1991), *A Short History of Ethics*, London, Routledge.

Marsh, S. and J. Soulsby (1990), *Outlines of English Law*, Berkshire, McGraw-Hill.

Mill, J. S. (1972), *Utilitarianism: On Liberty and Considerations on Representative Government*, ed. H. B. Acton, London, J. M. Dent.

Montgomery, J. (1993), Consent to health care for children, *Journal of Child Law*, V, pp. 117–24.

Mulholland, M. (1993), Re W (A Minor): autonomy, consent and the anorexic teenager, *Professional Negligence*, IX, pp. 21–4.

Murphy, J. (1992), W(h)ither adolescent autonomy?, *Journal of Social Welfare and Family Law*, VI, pp. 529–44.

NHS Management Executive (1992), *A Guide to Consent for Examination or Treatment*, London.

Nicholls, M. (1993), Consent to medical treatment, *Family Law*, 23, pp. 30–3.

Pappworth, M. H. (1967), *Human Guinea Pigs*, London, Routledge.

Paton, H. J. (1948), *The Moral Law*, London, Hutchinson.

Polit, D. F. and B. P. Hungler (1991), *Nursing Research: Principles and Methods*, 4th ed., Philadelphia, Lippincott.

Pyne, R. H. (1992), *Professional Discipline in Nursing, Midwifery and Health Visiting*, Oxford, Blackwell.

Rachels, J. (1986), *The End of Life*, Oxford, Oxford University Press.

Raphael, D. D. (1981), *Moral Philosophy*, Oxford, Oxford University Press.

Rawls, J. (1972), *A Theory of Justice*, Oxford, Oxford University Press.

Royal College of Nursing (1977), *Ethics Related to Research in Nursing*, London, RCN.

Royal College of Nursing (1992), *Seclusion, Control and Restraint in Hospitals and Units for the Mentally Disordered*, London, RCN.

Royal College of Physicians (1989), *Guidelines on the Practice of Ethics Committees on Research Involving Human Subjects*, 2nd ed., London, RCP.

Royal College of Physicians (1990), *Guidelines on Research on Healthy Volunteers*, London, RCP.

Royal Commission on Civil Liability and Compensation for Personal Injury (1978), *Report* (Cmnd 7054), London, HMSO.

Russell, B. (1992), *Why I Am Not A Christian*, London, Routledge.

Sheldon, S. (1993), 'Who is the mother to make the judgment?': The construction of woman in English abortion law, *Feminist Legal Studies*, I, pp. 3–22.

Singer, P. (1979), *Practical Ethics*, London, Routledge.

Singer, P. and D. Wells, (1984), *The Reproductive Revolution*, New York, Oxford University Press.

Smithells, R. W., S. Sheppard, C. J. Schorah, et al. (1976), Vitamin deficiencies and neural tube defects, *Archives in the Diseases of Childhood*, 51, pp. 944–50.

Stern, K. (1993), Court-ordered caesarian sections: in whose interests?, *Modern Law Review*, 56, pp. 238–43.

UKCC (1987), *Confidentiality*, London, UKCC.

UKCC (1989), *Exercising Accountability*, London, UKCC.

UKCC (1992a), *Code of Professional Conduct*, London, UKCC.

UKCC (1992b), *The Scope of Professional Practice*, London, UKCC.

Urwin, J. (1992), Re R: the resurrection of parental powers?, *Professional Negligence*, VIII, pp. 69–73.

Whitelaw, A. (1986), Death as an option in neonatal intensive care, *Lancet*, August 9, pp. 328–31.

Williams, A. (1985), The value of QUALYs, *Health and Social Service Journal*, 18 July.

Williams, G. (1985), The Gillick saga I and II, *New Law Journal*, 135, pp. 1156–8 and 1179–82.

Zander, M. (1990), *The Law Making Process*, London, Weidenfeld.

Index